CURING FATIGUE

A Step-by-Step Plan to Uncover and Eliminate the Causes of Chronic Fatigue

DAVID S. BELL, M.D.
Clinical instructor, Harvard Medical School
and STEF DONEV

Rodale Press, Emmaus, Pennsylvania

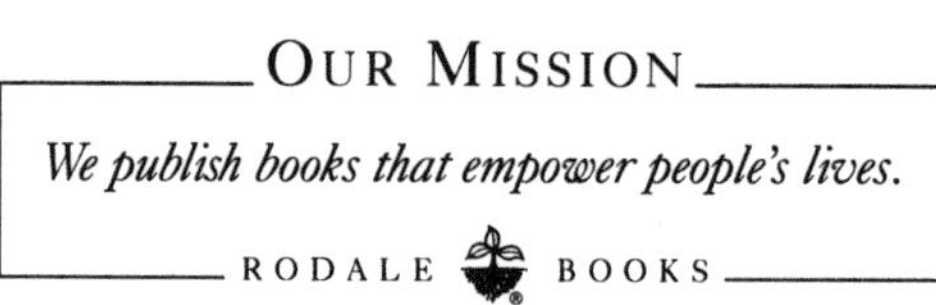

Printed in the United States of America on acid-free ∞, recycled paper containing a minimum of 20% post-consumer waste ♻

Cover designer: Lisa Nawaz

If you have any questions or comments concerning this book, please write:

Rodale Press
Book Readers' Service
33 East Minor Street
Emmaus, PA 18098

Library of Congress Cataloging-in-Publication Data

Bell, David S.
Curing fatigue : a step-by-step plan to uncover and eliminate the causes of chronic fatigue / by David S. Bell and Stef Donev.
p. cm.
Includes index.
ISBN 0-87596-161-4 : hardcover
1. Chronic fatigue syndrome. 2. Fatigue. I. Donev, Stef. II. Title.
RB150.F37B45 1993
616′.047—dc20 92-42786
CIP

Distributed in the book trade by St. Martin's Press

2 4 6 8 10 9 7 5 3 1 hardcover

NOTICE

This book is meant to supplement the advice and guidance of your physician. No two medical conditions are the same. What's more, medical treatment varies from region to region and is changing constantly. Therefore, we urge you to seek the best medical resources available to help you make informed decisions.

ABOUT THE AUTHORS

David S. Bell, M.D., is a graduate of Harvard University. He received his medical degree from Boston University and trained for five years as a pediatrics specialist, concentrating on chronic childhood diseases.

With his wife, Karen (an internist with special training in treatment of infectious diseases), Dr. Bell began to study an unusual illness that in 1985 became known as chronic Epstein-Barr virus syndrome, the so-called yuppie flu. After studying children affected in this epidemic, they presented evidence to an international conference in 1988 in Rome, Italy, proving that Epstein-Barr virus was not the cause of the illness.

Dr. Bell has continued researching this illness, now called chronic fatigue immune dysfunction syndrome (CFIDS), and is internationally recognized as an expert in the field. His book on CFIDS, *The Disease of a Thousand Names,* was published by Pollard Publications in 1991. Dr. Bell currently practices medicine in Cambridge, Massachusetts. He is on the faculty of Harvard Medical School and the staff of the Department of Pediatrics at Cambridge Hospital.

Stef Donev is an author, journalist and corporate communicator, and a former reporter for the *Toronto Star,* the Associated Press, the *London (Ontario) Free Press* and other newspapers in the United States and Canada. He frequently writes on medical, health and science matters and develops scripts for television, audiovisual and live presentations. His articles have appeared in *Today's Health, Urban Doctor, Newscience, Men's Health Quarterly, Cosmopolitan, TV Guide* and the *Washington Post.*

Donev's most recent book for Rodale Press is *20/20: A Total Guide to Improving Your Vision and Preventing Eye Disease,* written with Mitchell Friedlaender, M.D. Donev lives in Pine Mountain Club, California, with his wife and three children.

Contents

PART I THE NATURE OF FATIGUE

CHAPTER 1

There Is a Solution

Fatigue free!

It's a wonderful concept. But what does it mean?

Does it mean that you'll never be tired again? Never be physically or mentally exhausted? Never feel any sort of fatigue at all?

No. What it means is that being fatigued doesn't have to be anything more than a temporary condition.

You needn't feel constantly tired for the rest of your life. For that matter, you may not even have to feel that way for the rest of the week.

You can do something about it. You can replace fatigue with energy.

But to do it, you'll have to overcome a few obstacles. In the past, lack of interest among many physicians was one of the obstacles, but that may be changing.

TIRED? YES, AND WHAT ELSE?

Doctors are trained to treat illnesses. But throughout history, fatigue has been considered a *symptom* of an illness—not an illness in itself.

When you tell a doctor you are tired all the time, he or she is almost sure to ask, "And . . . what else?" The doctor needs more clues. That's why he turns to testing when tiredness coincides with other symptoms.

If you're tired all the time and you also have a pain at Point A and get Test Results B, well, then maybe you have the disease on page 128 of the doctor's medical book. If you're tired all the time and have discomfort at Point C and get Test Results D, then maybe you have the disease on page 347.

But if all you are is tired all the time, who's to say what's wrong with you? Tiredness is a natural basic body response, and pinpointing it as a singular disease in itself is usually beyond the reach of simple diagnostic tools.

Doctors know of hundreds of medical conditions that have fatigue as a symptom. For that reason, merely knowing fatigue is present in your case rarely helps the physician to tell you why it's there.

While some doctors do approach the subject of fatigue directly, most tend to shrug their shoulders as if to say, "That's life." They might give you some general advice about reducing stress, taking it easier at work, cutting down on drinking and so forth, but usually that's as far as they go.

We hope to do better. In this book, my coauthor, Stef Donev, and I consider fatigue both as a symptom and as an illness. We also look at what fatigue is, the different forms it takes and the many medical, psychological and environmental conditions that can cause it.

YOU CAN SNAP OUT OF IT

We provide tips and techniques that can be used to erase or at least ease fatigue, plus we share inspiring case studies of people who have experienced different types of chronic fatigue and have come through feeling vigorous again.

At the end of the book we present the 30-Day High-Energy Program: a way to examine and evaluate your own life and to find out what diets and activities might affect your well-being and energy levels.

But this book is to be used in conjunction with, not as a substitute for, a complete medical checkup. The systematic approach, the steps you must take to end your fatigue, will have to be based on the results of a thorough medical evaluation. It does little good to work on stress reduction if the real reason you are tired is an overactive thyroid gland. Cutting out caffeine may do wonders for your nerves, but it won't do anything to relieve exhaustion if you are walking around with an undiagnosed disease that's draining your vitality.

Also, we urge you not to flip to the 30-Day High-Energy Program without reading the first part of the book. Parts I and II contain important information to help you make the most of that program.

We're suggesting approaches here that have to do with overall changes. These are not quick-fix measures that won't work or last.

WHAT DOES FATIGUE MEAN TO YOU?

First, let's talk about fatigue itself. One of the main problems a doctor has in dealing with fatigue is defining exactly what it means to the complaining patient.

Ask four people to talk about the fatigue they feel in their lives, and you are quite likely to get four decidedly different answers.

- "Well, Doctor, I had a pretty good day. Best day I've had in months. For the past week or so I've been able to get by on only ten hours of sleep a night and two short naps a day: an hour after breakfast and two more hours after lunch. On Tuesday I was actually able to vacuum the house, load the dishwasher and even sort some of the laundry."
- "Gee, Doctor, I don't know what's wrong with me. I was only 21 miles into the marathon Thursday, and I totally pooped out. I barely made the last 5 miles. I finished seventh out of a field of 983. And it was only my third marathon this month. My body is betraying me! What can I do to get my energy back? This fatigue thing is really scary."
- "Is my energy level getting better? What difference does it make? What difference does anything make? I think I'd rather sleep through my life than have to be awake for it. It would be a lot better that way. But as it is, I'm up all night. Can't you give me some stronger sleeping pills?"
- "What a week. The baby is teething, keeping us both up all night. The city's putting in a new sewer line on our street. They

start work at 7:00 A.M. And the phone! The newspaper made a mistake in an ad for a new pizza parlor—they listed our number! We're zombies! I fell asleep over my cereal bowl this morning—until the jackhammer started outside. But we're leaving the baby with my mother this weekend and going to a quiet motel to sleep for 48 hours. We'll be fine on Monday."

The first patient's energy expectations are so low that any day requiring less than 14 hours of sleep and allowing even a little work to get done is a good one.

The marathon runner's expectations for stamina are absurdly and dangerously high. To this person, even the thought of taking a rest is a sign of weakness, and the very idea of feeling tired is considered an act of betrayal by the body.

The third patient is so lost in depression that nothing matters. Fatigue is hardly a relevant factor in this case.

The parent of the teething baby knows what's wrong and exactly how to solve the problem—and is making plans to do it.

Are all four suffering from fatigue? By your definition, probably not. But by theirs . . . yes.

Unlike cancer, diabetes or a broken arm, the medical definition of fatigue is elusive, and the objective signs almost invite misinterpretation. So let's start off with the meanings of some basic terms to make sure we all agree on what's being discussed.

The verb *to tire* means to exhaust or greatly decrease physical strength. It implies a draining of one's strength. If you just ran a race or moved 500 pounds of shingles, if you spent a day keeping up with a three-year-old or stayed awake most of last night—you're tired! Your supply of energy is gone.

The word *fatigue,* used in a physical sense, refers to the condition of cells or organs that have undergone excessive activity resulting in the loss of power or capacity to respond to stimulation. As you can see, *fatigue* implies that you and your body have gone beyond being merely *tired.*

If you wake up after two hours of sleep and you can't get going, you're tired. But if you sleep a full eight hours or more and still can't get through the day and do a *reasonable* amount of work, you're fatigued. And if this happens day after day, then you have chronic fatigue.

LISTEN TO YOUR BODY

It doesn't do any good to say that there is no reason for this fatigue, that you get enough sleep, eat well and take care of yourself. The body does not lie. When your body is chronically fatigued, something is wrong, either medically, emotionally or psychologically. It's as simple as that.

Some people suffer from unrelenting fatigue simply because they insist upon pushing themselves too far. "But I shouldn't be tired" is a story that doctors hear all too often. "I get four hours of sleep a night, and that's all a person needs."

Says who?

"Says me. And my father—four hours was enough for him. Anyone who claims to need more is lazy and slothful, he used to say. Besides, I'm a busy person. Busy, busy, busy! I have a lot of things that must be done. Important things. And I can't afford to be tired. So give me some pills. Fix me."

If this is your attitude, maybe it's up to you to do the fixing. Ask yourself whether your tiredness is actually due to a medical or psychological problem or simply a lack of self-care. Of course, if it's the latter, you may soon be faced with a medical or psychological problem as a result of your carelessness. Evaluate this possibility thoroughly. The answer could be a lifesaver.

One of the first areas to investigate in your search for the root of your fatigue is sleep habits. How much sleep do you get, how good is it, and is it natural or drug induced? Stress is another major consideration. And after that comes depression.

Among the other areas to look at for clues to your chronic fatigue: your diet, your general health, your job, your relationships, the medication you take, your drinking, how much you smoke. The list goes on and on. Any or all of these can cause and contribute to fatigue.

But there are different types of fatigue: chronic fatigue, which means you feel tired all the time; and the fatigue disease, chronic fatigue immune dysfunction syndrome, usually referred to as CFIDS (pronounced *CEE-fids* and sometimes called chronic fatigue syndrome, or CFS).

There are two major differences between ordinary chronic fatigue and CFIDS.

First: severity. To be recognized as a victim of CFIDS, a person has to experience a 50 percent loss of activity over a six-month period, and the onset of fatigue must be new and traceable to that period, not an extension of some previous bout with fatigue.

Second: the pattern of symptoms. People can be chronically fatigued but have no other symptoms; they just feel tired all the time. CFIDS victims display patterns of other coincidental symptoms, which we'll consider in the coming chapters.

IS IT YOUR LIFESTYLE?

Medical doctors know, as do most laypeople, that fatigue can be linked to specific actions and physical and psychological conditions, such as athletics, carbohydrate craving, commuting, computing, drinking, drugging, jet lag, menopause, migraines, excessive noise, PMS, retirement and shift work, to name but a few. Since these types of fatigue result from specific conditions or circumstances, changing the condition usually eliminates the fatigue. The complications set in when there is more than one fatigue-causing complaint—and that's usually the case.

Suppose, for example, you say you are tired all the time because you don't get enough sleep. But if you also need to lose 100 pounds, and you smoke, drink too much and suffer from migraines, plus you spend three hours a day stuck in traffic and you live next to a musician who practices the tuba while you're trying to sleep, it's obvious that moving to a quieter apartment will solve only some of your problems. You have other concerns to deal with before you can expect your fatigue to disappear. But, as you'll see later, these various causes of your fatigue can be isolated and dealt with.

MILLIONS OF PEOPLE ARE TIRED AND DON'T KNOW WHY

No one really knows how many people suffer from chronic fatigue. But a recent study of the records of one medical clinic showed that 20 percent of all the adults being treated there (for a wide variety of ills) said they were also plagued with persistent fatigue so intense that it interfered with their daily activities.

These findings surprised many physicians. The medical community is only beginning to realize just how big a problem chronic fatigue is.

Some chronic fatigue sufferers actually were born that way. They have been tired all their lives. They don't know what it's like *not* to feel tired. But the vast majority of those afflicted with chronic fatigue started out with the regular supply of energy and vitality. Then, over the years, it was somehow eaten away—by such things as illness, depression, work, relationships, diet, environment and a host of other factors.

Even worse, many people accept this never-ending fatigue as normal. Exhausted and barely able to drag themselves through the day, they find life to be a struggle to survive.

The problem is compounded for those who consider their fatigue a sign of personal weakness or failure. They don't know what's wrong, but whatever it is, they are sure that it's their fault. As a result, they're afraid to talk about it because of what people might think of them.

But when these people do finally open up and seek help, all their complaints are basically the same: no energy, no pep, washed out and exhausted all the time. Simple tasks such as housecleaning, preparing dinner, playing with the children or going off to work seem to require much more energy than they can muster. Fatigue dominates every aspect of their lives, from the momentous to the mundane.

One of the worst things about having chronic fatigue is that you might not realize just how tired you are and just how much of your life—as well as your potential for life—you are missing. Why? Because chronic fatigue develops gradually. You don't wake up one morning suddenly aware that you're suffering from chronic fatigue.

It might be compared to the onset of frostbite: What starts as an annoying tingle in cheeks and nose exposed to bitter winter cold slowly becomes an ache you determine to bear until you get where you're going. But by the time you arrive, you no longer feel the pain. All feeling is gone, and damage to your skin may be severe.

The same kind of thing can happen with chronic fatigue. You may wind up missing or ruining some of the best years of your life without even knowing it—and possibly damage the lives of others at the same time.

But that scenario isn't inevitable. There are solutions to constant feelings of tiredness, and you do have choices. You can break out of the cycle.

HOW TO USE THIS BOOK

Fatigue has numerous faces, and we describe and discuss many of them in these pages. Along with the medical facts, you will find a series of case studies that tell of people who suffered from and dealt with their own cases of fatigue. But remember, it's unlikely that any case study will be exactly like your story. Each battle with fatigue is unique. So when you read these histories, focus on the similarities. That's where you will find the solutions you can apply to yourself. You will see that often the various components of fatigue may respond to simple remedies, some that you can offer yourself and others your doctor can provide.

You may have to make some difficult choices in changing the way you live so you can begin to enjoy your life again. That will take determination and hard work.

A nagging voice in the back of your brain may try to convince you that nothing will change, that nothing will help, that you might as well give up. But your life *will* change if you work at it. And you will regain your freedom—freedom from fatigue; freedom to be fully alive.

CHAPTER

2

Why You're Tired

Millions of people are tired all the time, but they don't know why. They don't even have a clue. Their small store of energy doesn't allow sorting through the multitude of potential causes to pinpoint what's sapping their strength and sucking the joy out of life.

Others do know the cause of their problem, but they won't seek or accept medical or psychological help, nor will they make the lifestyle changes necessary to solve the problem. They may be smokers, heavy drinkers or drug abusers. They may eat poorly, skip sleep or push themselves too hard. In some cases, they're so emotionally tied to another person that they no longer have a life of their own.

Regardless of what makes them feel so tired, they must care enough to take *some* sort of action. They must come to a point reached by a character played some years ago by Peter Finch in the movie *Network:* "I'm mad as hell and I'm not going to take it anymore!"

In other words, when you're finally sick and tired of being sick and tired, you will actually do something about it.

But what can you do? Where do you start? How do you go about regaining your lost energy?

TOO FATIGUED TO FLEX

Even if you have the best-developed muscles in the world, fatigue can make you as weak as a kitten. Fatigue saps your strength, not your musculature. So having a great body drained of all energy is like having a high-powered sports car that's out of gas.

There are a lot of muscles—approximately 650 of them—each a bundle of individual fibers. Muscles range in size from the minuscule ones attached to the tiny bones of your inner ear to the massive gluteus maximus in your buttocks.

All muscles really do is contract and relax. That's why many of them are paired. Your biceps, for example, do nothing except pull your forearm up. The bulge you feel when you flex your biceps is just that—your biceps. It gets thicker when it contracts. To straighten your arm again you have to contract your triceps, the muscle at the back of your upper arm. If you had a muscle spasm that contracted both your biceps and triceps at once, your arm would either remain frozen in position or move spastically.

Whatever muscles you use, the power all comes from the same source, the energy stored in cells in the form of adenosine triphosphate (ATP). If the energy isn't there, or if something interferes with its release, your muscles can't work.

Everything you do—from running a race to swallowing your dinner to rolling over in bed—requires muscles. For instance, it takes more than 30 facial muscles to control everything from blinking and moving your eyes to chewing—and smiling. (Those interested in conserving energy should note that it takes fewer muscles to smile than to frown.) The muscular

You'll probably have to figure most of it out for yourself. Few physicians have the patience or time to sort through the many potential causes of your particular tiredness, but *you* do. After all, it is your body and your life. With the right approach and a little study, you'll see many avenues of treatment open up.

EVERYDAY FATIGUE VS. ABNORMAL FATIGUE

Because there are so many types of fatigue, the search becomes easier if you divide fatigue into two categories: *everyday* and *abnormal.*

system forms an intricate maze beneath the skin; it's a high-speed highway that carries commands from the brain to the various parts of the body that obey them.

Let's say that you want to greet someone. Here's the simplified version of what your brain tells your body so you can shake hands.

1. Turn to face the other person.
2. Extend your upper arm, forearm and hand.
3. Make sure your fingers are straight and in the right position to shake hands.
4. When the other person's hand meets yours, grasp it.
5. Shake the hand.
6. Release the hand.
7. Drop your upper arm, forearm and hand to your side.

While going through all of this, you probably want to nod your head and offer a pleasant and friendly smile, too. Also, you want to be sure you use the right amount of force. You want to extend your arm, not punch the person, and you want to shake his hand, not crush it.

To do all that, your brain has to send a series of commands through your spinal column and motor nerves. There are separate commands to every cell involved in each motion, and there's a different command for each function that each muscle must perform. One command initiates an action, another one ends it.

Luckily, you don't have to go through that thought process every time you want to shake hands. All you have to do is decide to shake hands and let the brain and nervous system take over, so you can concentrate on what you're going to say during the greeting.

Think of everyday fatigue as the type that results from heavy exercise, a hectic schedule, lack of sleep, poor nutrition, air pollution and the temporary emotional jolts that accompany life's lower moments. There is no way you can avoid all of these factors permanently and still be part of the modern world and the human race. They are simply the stuff of life. (Some researchers include smoking, obesity, drinking and excessive stress as causes of everyday fatigue.) While these circumstances do not necessarily cause tremendous fatigue by themselves, they certainly do contribute to it. And if they become major factors in your everyday life, they can make themselves major causes of abnormal fatigue.

Only you can determine what your fatigue factors are and how much of your life they steal from you. Then you can develop a strategy for battling them. To do that, you must assess the details of your life, your experiences and your emotions and try to relate them to your symptoms. It will take time and effort, particularly when it comes to dealing with the greatest obstacle of all in the war against fatigue—apathy.

Apathy is the source of that negative litany sure to interfere with taking any real action to overcome chronic fatigue: "I'll start tomorrow," "One of these days . . ." "What's the use?" "What difference does it make?" "This won't work; it's a waste of time."

But you can do what it takes, and it will be worth the effort. If you don't succeed right away, don't be discouraged. The program in this book aims for slow, steady and lasting improvement, not fireworks that flare up and quickly die out.

Remember that fatigue is the enemy, not you. Be gentle and kind to yourself, but be firm. Make realistic plans and resolutions, and carry them out.

At the end of this book you'll find an easy-to-follow plan for such an approach, the 30-Day High-Energy Program. But before you can follow it, you have to know exactly what saps the energy you're losing.

BREAKDOWNS IN THE POWER LINE

When the energy pathway is disrupted, the symptoms suggest where the power chain has been broken. For example, if there is a problem with digestion, the beginning of the cycle, basic general energy needed for our many body functions is reduced. This shows up as overall fatigue and weight loss. However, if the disruption is near the end of the chain—say, lack of energy to contract a muscle—the cause might be some specific, localized weakness but relatively little generalized fatigue.

So when a person complains of all-around fatigue, it could be due to a fundamental dietary disruption (difficult to trace because so many factors are involved) or to something such as an illness that drains massive amounts of energy as quickly as the body produces it.

Think about getting energy from food the way you get heat from a fireplace. As the fire burns, you sense and enjoy the light and warmth (the energy) released from the wood.

Some heat sources, such as furnaces or water heaters, have a mechanism designed to store heat for later use. In a similar way, your body allows you to process food and store the energy released from it. When the system is working properly and you need the energy hours after eating a meal, you simply tap your body's storage sites.

In a perfectly designed system, energy is released in a steady flow without wide variations. But we must have reserves to meet sudden additional demands. And once an emergency has been met, the energy-release system must return to a steady, constant comfort level.

THE SIX BASIC CAUSES OF FATIGUE

As with any system, problems can develop. When it comes to our energy system, there are six basic potential trouble spots.

1. Stress and emotions
2. Depression
3. Medical illness
4. Chronic fatigue immune dysfunction syndrome (CFIDS)
5. Sleep disorders
6. Poor nutrition

Experts usually agree on the six basic causes but not always on which one is the most important. A lot depends upon the type of fatigue you experience. Are you always tired? Tired most of the time, or just now and then? Do you feel you need a nap at some specific time of day? Are you already wiped out when you get to work or before you even tackle the dishes in the sink? Do you get that tired feeling as soon as you know you have a meeting with the boss or when your long-winded neighbor calls? Are you usually on the verge of collapse a half hour before dinner—or a half hour after?

There you are—different types of tiredness; the various times, situations and ways they might strike; and, of course, their different causes.

You will notice specific patterns in your tiredness as you examine the six primary causes. Use these patterns as guidelines as you search for solutions to your own low-energy problems. Each of the causes has its own chapter later in the book.

HOW WE PRODUCE ENERGY FOR THE BODY ELECTRIC

The sole purpose of your body, a machine that was issued to you in the womb, is to carry the conscious, spiritual and intellectual you through life. To do that, it needs food it can convert into energy. The type and amount of food it gets helps determine the quantity and quality of that energy, which, in turn, influences the length and quality of your life.

Here's a brief look at how food converts to energy, how we put that energy to work and how fatigue is often an indication of a problem or breakdown in the food/energy/work cycle. (The word *energy,* from the Greek word *energia,* "in-work," means the capacity to do work. If you have energy, you can do work; without it, you can't.)

Since your body stores its own energy supplies, it is, in effect, a battery—a rechargeable one, at that! Using protein enzymes as the basic tools, the body converts food into the energy it stores and uses.

The enzymes go to work as soon as food enters your body. Enzymes are catalysts; they change things without being changed themselves. Hundreds of types of enzymes do different jobs as part of your digestive system. Like a robot on an assembly line, each performs a specific job on every item as it goes by. But while each item is altered in some way, the robots remain the same.

Protein enzymes initiate a series of chemical reactions in your digestive system. After each reaction, the energy-producing substance taken from your food is passed on to the next step in the cycle.

All the many types of foods that you eat are broken down by the enzymes into three basic compounds: carbohydrates become glucose, or sugar; proteins become amino acids; and fats dissolve to become fatty acids. These compounds are absorbed by your body's cells, and there they are further broken down into a complex chemical compound known as acetyl coenzyme A, or simply acetyl CoA. Then comes the indispensable ingredient, oxygen.

Without oxygen life is impossible, not only because we need it for breathing, but also because it is necessary for transforming acetyl CoA into essential body energy. That transformation takes place in rod-shaped bodies called mitochondria, contained in the cells. The oxygen and acetyl CoA are combined in a process called the Krebs cycle, which involves about 20 different steps and turns us on, so to speak.

The body's "battery system" consists of a unique sugar solution that holds and stores high-energy phosphate bonds. This solution is called adenosine diphosphate, or ADP, when the battery is empty. (It is diphosphate because each molecule contains two phosphate atoms.) When oxygen and acetyl CoA combine to make a high-energy bond, a third phosphate atom is added to the ADP molecule, forming adenosine triphosphate (ATP). With that third atom, the battery is energized, and the energy is stored for later use.

ATP is probably the single most important chemical we have in us. It is also the end product of the human body's sophisticated yet surprisingly simple process of reducing the food we eat to its component parts, then extracting and storing the energy they contain.

Since the ATP is a battery, its energy capacity can be measured in terms of moles, the common scientific unit of measurement for complex molecules. (Each mole contains more than 1,000 calories of potential energy.) When this energy is used up in running the body machinery, the drained battery is left with only ADP until more acetyl CoA combines with oxygen to produce the third phosphate atom, the high-energy bond, and the ADP once again becomes ATP. The process—ADP to ATP to ADP—continues as long as you live.

ATP is involved in nearly every body process. It takes part in building proteins and enzymes in the liver and is required to supply the energy for the work your muscles do. (See "Too Fatigued to Flex" on page 12.) ATP also plays a role in transmitting impulses along the nerves. It regulates the opening and closing of the gates that lead to and from each cell, allowing every cell in your body to absorb or discharge various elements and compounds. ATP is even used to produce more ATP.

This is all part of the body's magnificent natural process for producing its own energy to keep itself going.

How Our Food Is Transformed into Energy

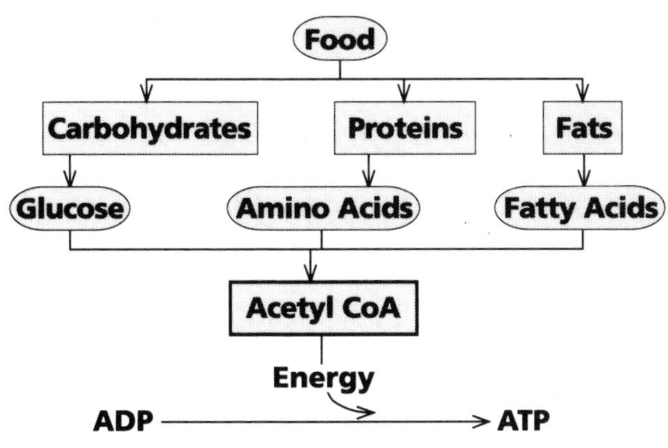

Stress and emotions. Stress is as much a part of living as breathing is, and it's not all bad. In fact, a certain amount of stress is necessary—it keeps us sharp and on our toes. But stress and other emotional conditions can and do use up a lot of energy. And when overpowered by stress, the body shuts down just like a household fuse or a circuit breaker, and we become apathetic, burned-out and exhausted.

The task lies in learning how to manage those stresses instead of letting them manage you. Like blood pressure and body temperature, emotions exist within each of us and can be read and measured, analyzed and sorted through. But that takes time and an objective view of our own emotional state.

Depression. Even though depression is an emotional condition, it can be debilitating and can lead to so much self-destructive behavior that it deserves special attention. Serious clinical depression requires professional intervention.

Medical illness. More than 200 medical illnesses are associated with tiredness or fatigue. They range from common allergies, such as hay fever, all the way up to cancer and multiple sclerosis. It is important to remember that if you are sick, your body needs more rest. Pushing yourself just aggravates the illness and adds to your fatigue.

Chronic fatigue immune dysfunction syndrome (CFIDS). Over the years CFIDS has been known as everything from yuppie flu to antibody negative lupus. All in all, it's had more than 50 different names in the past 30 years, but until recently most physicians simply called it chronic fatigue syndrome (CFS).

For some time CFIDS was mistakenly identified as chronic Epstein-Barr virus syndrome. The British, who call it myalgic encephalomyelitis, have been studying this illness for almost 40 years. CFIDS causes a severe and persistent fatigue that, combined with a specific pattern of other symptoms, stretches for months or years on end. It was first discussed in the modern medical literature of the United States in 1935.

Sleep disorders. It's remarkable that this common cause of fatigue is often overlooked. Theoretically its role is quite logical: You're tired because you don't sleep well or long enough. But pinpointing the reasons for your sleep disturbance may not be so easy. It might be due to a simple cause such as too much noise or light, or a sleep disorder such as sleep apnea or narcolepsy.

In some cases insomnia is a by-product of another condition, perhaps a bladder problem that requires getting up frequently during the night to go to the bathroom. Excessive drinking can also contribute to poor sleep, as can reliance on drugs, including sleeping pills.

Sleep-related fatigue is usually secondary to known problems with sleep and is second or third on the list of symptoms.

Poor nutrition. This problem can be insidious and often difficult to pinpoint. Chronic fatigue is caused by *too much* food more often than by too little. Obese people use up excessive amounts of energy in carrying their increased body weight.

Other nutritional disorders include vitamin and mineral imbalances leading to medical conditions such as anemia. But while nutritional and medical disorders often overlap, poor nutrition is usually the culprit behind fatigue. Food allergies can also be a major factor in chronic fatigue.

Now you know why your personal input is essential in getting to the bottom of your fatigue problem. Of course, your doctor can help, through testing and experience, to uncover the mysteries in your body that explain your lack of vigor. But only you can describe the events, sensations and reactions that have affected you over the months and years and might reveal the reason for the drain on that most precious reserve—energy.

CHAPTER 3

The High Costs of Dysfunctional Fatigue

Imagine being so tired every day that you were unable to go to work. Suppose the fatigue persisted; you'd soon lose your job and it would be hard for you to find another. That kind of situation would put a real price tag on your own chronic fatigue.

Fortunately, most of us who are tired all the time can make it to work, do our jobs and then go home. But because we do manage somehow, the price we pay for our own personal degree of fatigue is much harder to compute. Of course, being constantly tired—or even being tired most of the time—takes its toll in promotions, bonuses and chances at more interesting assignments. We do our jobs by the numbers and lose the initiative, the interest, the pride and the sense of accomplishment that make a job more than just a paycheck. And merely showing up isn't enough to guarantee job security. An employer isn't impressed by a worker who acts like a zombie, loses track of conversations, is the last to respond during a meeting or generally seems to be a few steps behind everyone else.

The workplace is only one area that exacts a price for our chronic fatigue. When we come home tired, our chores, recreation and personal relationships also suffer. Is anything more frustrating than being unable to participate in your own life?

Outside the home, friends, bill collectors, teammates and teachers don't care to hear that you're tired. They presume that you'll perform as usual. They don't understand about the types and degrees of fatigue and the many possible causes. If you're tired, they expect you to snap out of it, just as they often do. If you don't or can't, you pay the penalty in diminished status. The idea that your exhaustion could be a full-blown disease—chronic fatigue immune dysfunction syndrome (CFIDS)—is absurd to most people.

Yet some researchers estimate that two million people in the United States are out of work because of CFIDS alone. If that figure is correct, it means a direct loss of nearly $600 billion from the nation's economy. That figure does not include the financial aid to those forced to apply for welfare or some other form of financial or social assistance.

THE PLEASURES OF HIGH ENERGY

There's nothing like a feeling of healthy energy when it comes to taking joy in every day. With energy, everything seems possible. Hopes soar and work becomes pleasurable, productive and satisfying.

Every type of fatigue—in fact, each individual case of fatigue—carries its own price tag. Like CFIDS, those price tags have personal as well as nationwide economic consequences.

When you have that energetic good feeling, what do you do with it? How do you make it pay off in your life?

Maybe you go dancing, learn how to scuba dive, spend time playing with the kids or grandchildren, take a class, go for walks, start and stick with an exercise program, become active in a club or group or become more involved in the world around you.

But if you get tired a lot, you're limited and it shows in the way you live your life. You might have the drive and determination to start a class or a project but lack the energy to see it through. One day you're up and ready for anything; the next day you can barely get out of bed. Eventually you stop initiating projects because you know you won't have what it takes to follow up.

If your fatigue is truly severe, just holding a job or keeping a family together is a struggle. Life is an insurmountable mountain, and despair creeps in. All outside interests disappear. Simple tasks become drudgery. Now the controlling thought of daily life has become "What's the use? Why even try?"

To you fatigue may seem to be the most important thing blocking your contentment in life, but the apathy, despair and loss of self-esteem that can come with unrelenting exhaustion are even more important.

Think of it this way. A runner may work hard and train to achieve a personal goal—let's say doing five miles in 40 minutes. When the goal is finally met, the runner is wiped out but happy. The exhaustion is accepted, even welcome proof of the accomplishment.

Now consider a shift worker who feels exhausted from trying to maintain a nighttime work schedule and a normal daytime family life. To him, this tiredness is not the result of accomplishment. Instead, it is likely to be the first sign of progressive difficulties and despair, coupled with constant misgivings and thoughts of quitting.

As you can see, fatigue itself is not the critical factor. It is the way the fatigue relates to an acceptable quality of life that counts. If you experience tiredness in the course of living a life you enjoy, it is a reasonable price to pay, but if fatigue only corrodes your joy in life, the cost is too high.

When you're miserable because you're tired, your family and friends, employer and fellow workers will comment on the change in you. They will urge you to deal with your problem. If the tiredness continues too long, their care and concern may turn into anger and resentment. In their eyes, you no longer have a problem—you *are* a problem. They wonder if you really don't want to feel energetic enough to work or be active.

If you accept the idea that you are lazy, your self-esteem plummets along with your energy and ability to work. You might ignore the possibility that a medical problem exists and decide to deal with your "laziness" instead. But that won't get to the root of the problem. Instead you'll simply repeat endless cycles of lost self-esteem, tiredness, apathy and depression.

All it takes to trigger this syndrome is losing enough energy to make a noticeable change in your life and your lifestyle—especially if those changes affect other people. The fatigue might not even seem severe to you, so be on the lookout for the signs.

FATIGUE CAN FLATTEN RELATIONSHIPS

Lacking energy and being tired all the time can spoil more than your pleasure in life. It can also damage your relationships—even kill them.

Relationships are based on and nurtured by communication between the parties. But communicating takes effort. You have to listen carefully, feel what the other person is thinking and experiencing, transfer yourself to that person's perspective and show compassion. You also have to show up for dates and group activities and be a true, enthusiastic participant.

As your energy level goes down, these duties become increasingly difficult to fulfill. The tiredness may persist or escalate to a point where it becomes impossible to accomplish these actions. And while it is nice to say that love conquers all, love usually needs some energetic help to do so.

Chronically tired people don't have the energy to socialize. They can't concentrate long enough to hear about somebody else's problems because it takes all they've got to think about their own. They can't get excited about anything, let alone someone else's good fortune. No wonder their relationships tend to become clouded with misunderstandings and impatience.

Explanations such as "I'm too tired" are ignored or elicit an angry response from intimates: "No one can be that tired all the time!"

Suspicions arise; communication comes to a virtual halt. Depression and apathy set in. It's the familiar vicious cycle. More than one marriage or friendship has collapsed because one or both parties were just too tired to keep it going.

DON'T BANKRUPT YOUR LIFE

We have seen that being tired all of the time is expensive in terms of money, personal and professional growth, group and private relationships, life enjoyment and self-esteem. You don't have to have a severe case of CFIDS to suffer this way. Even a 10 or 15 percent loss in energy levels can cause costly, long-lasting consequences.

When you're tired all the time, you can even lose track of what "normal" energy really is. Just how active is an active life supposed to be? How much rest is enough?

At a certain point you forget how much energy you once had. The fatigue that started out as a minor hindrance has evolved into a seemingly insurmountable obstacle that prevents you from reaching ordinary goals. Eventually even the goals disappear.

To regain your lost energy, be realistic. Then figure out just what you are striving for, and devise a realistic plan to achieve it. The next chapter will launch you into your program.

CHAPTER 4

How Tired Are You Really?

For months now you've refused dinner invitations from close friends, passed on outings with the kids, said no to sex with your mate—in fact, you've given up just about every activity you used to enjoy. Your explanation is always the same: You're tired. A lot of us feel that way from time to time, but we manage to keep up with friends and family. Why can't you? Are you overworked, tense, lazy or ill? Do you have a genuine chronic fatigue problem? And if you do, how serious is that problem? Let's find out.

We'll start by looking at four factors concerning your fatigue: its relative importance among other symptoms, plus the degree of your tiredness, the type of fatigue you feel and the way it limits your activity. These variables can supply hints to help you figure out why you are so tired.

IS IT "CAN'T" OR "DON'T WANT TO"?

Suppose you're asked to take part in a five-mile walkathon. If you can say yes right off, it's a pretty safe bet that you have no problem with chronic fatigue. If your answer is no, then maybe you do—and maybe you don't—have a problem. Are you saying no because you are too busy? Do you have a bad ankle? Are you overweight and out of shape? Do you tend to get headaches when you exercise? Would you just rather stay home and watch TV?

Or are you afraid that you'll pass out before you finish the course? Before you get halfway—or even get to the starting line?

If your refusal comes out of personal preferences or time commitments, you don't have a fatigue problem. However, if your answer is based upon doubts about your ability simply to accomplish the walk at all, you may be one of millions of people who are forced to schedule their activities around limited energy reserves. Their commitments are dictated by what absolutely must be accomplished; anything that can be managed beyond that is a luxury.

But how can you tell if your fatigue is normal or excessive? Here is a simple rule of thumb: If you're preoccupied by fatigue, something is wrong. Healthy people seldom think about fatigue. They don't have to. If they feel tired, they stop and take a breath or give themselves a short break. They know they'll be able to resume the activity in minutes.

If you do have chronic fatigue, the next step is to find out why. Remedies for a low energy level depend heavily on its specific cause.

RANK FATIGUE AMONG YOUR SYMPTOMS

Consider all of your medical symptoms and decide where chronic fatigue fits in. For example, if you have rheumatoid arthritis, the primary symptom on your list is probably joint pain, then comes morning stiffness, followed by difficulty in grasping small objects and, finally, tiredness.

Here are some more examples that show where chronic fatigue ranks among the symptoms of some other common complaints.

Sleep Disorders

1. Waking unrefreshed
2. Habitual snoring
3. Chronic fatigue
4. Sore throat
5. Daytime sleeping

Medical Illness

1. Frequent urination
2. Excessive thirst
3. Blurring vision
4. Yeast infections
5. Chronic fatigue

Chronic Fatigue Immune Dysfunction Syndrome (CFIDS)

1. Chronic fatigue
2. Headache
3. Muscle pain
4. Joint pain
5. Lymph node pain

Poor Nutrition

1. Weight changes
2. Dermatitis (rough skin, for example)
3. Chronic fatigue
4. Digestive disturbances
5. Thinning hair

Emotionally Based Problems

1. Stress or depression
2. Chronic fatigue
3. Headache
4. Abdominal pain
5. Weight changes

DIFFERENT DEGREES OF FATIGUE

Fatigue can be mild for one person and severe for another, then change from day to day. This guide will help you gauge the degree of your own fatigue.

Mild. You are tired at certain times of almost every day, usually in the morning or early afternoon. This feeling does not limit your overall activity, but you do have to adjust to it. You learn never to schedule an event or to count on accomplishing anything important or complicated during your "tired time."

YOUR PERSONAL TIREDNESS PATTERN

To determine your tiredness pattern, answer these questions and refer to the chart on page 31. Is your fatigue:

1. Mild? Does it affect only certain activities and only certain times of the day? Yes ____ No ____
2. Moderate? Are all activities affected? Does tiredness persist throughout the day, causing you to alter your plans? Yes ____ No ____
3. Severe? Are you always tired? Does fatigue cause a major disruption of your life? Yes ____ No ____

If you're at home, you should plan to put your feet up and relax at this time of day. If you're at work, you should try to avoid important conferences or critical private appointments during these hours.

So many people are tired at about 10:00 A.M. and 3:00 P.M. that Muzak—the company that pipes music into millions of homes and elevators around the world—plays faster music at these times as part of a calculated effort to stimulate listeners. These periods are known and accepted as times of low productivity around the world.

Few people pay much attention to this type of tiredness because it doesn't persist and doesn't really interfere with work. Fortunately, it is both the most common and the easiest to treat.

Moderate. You feel as you would on the last day of a very bad cold. You're not really sick anymore, but you're not quite healthy, either. You sense a nagging, persistent fatigue that you can't seem to shake.

While you can maintain a relatively normal schedule, you can't make plans to do much else. Chances are that when you've done your work for the day, you won't have the energy or ambition to do anything more strenuous than operate the remote control on the TV.

This degree of tiredness calls for medical attention.

Severe. You usually wake up exhausted, and you know you won't feel any better after you get up. Fatigue is the most compelling and important element of your day. After struggling through a few activities, you nearly always fall back into bed exhausted.

There are few, if any, moments when you experience any real physical power. Work is probably impossible, and your social life may be nonexistent.

It's a life reduced to the bare essentials! If an action doesn't contribute directly to your basic survival, you don't bother doing it.

Not only is this degree of fatigue the most difficult to overcome, it is also the most difficult to treat. It is often a by-product of medical illness. Severe fatigue is not limited to CFIDS sufferers, and it commonly requires serious medical intervention.

SORTING IT ALL OUT

Just as no two snowflakes are exactly the same, every case of chronic fatigue is different. We can use these differences to help determine what causes fatigue and how to treat it.

A patient named John is a case in point. John has diabetes mellitus, chronic anxiety, multiple allergies and a relatively mild case of CFIDS. Each of these conditions can bring on a different type of fatigue, and John can tell which fatigue is caused by which ailment. As a result, he is able to do what is necessary to get relief. For example, one type of tiredness tells John that his blood sugar level is higher than it should be, so he adjusts his medication accordingly and his energy rises. Another type tells him that one or more of his allergies is acting up, and he knows what action to take. CFIDS and chronic anxiety also produce specific types of fatigue, and each one has its own treatment.

Unfortunately, few people are as observant as John, so they often give up the effort to pinpoint and deal with their type of chronic fatigue.

Here are some hints that make fatigue identification easier.

Simple tiredness. You just want to sit and catch your breath for an hour or so; you're sure that then you'll be fine. You also know that you can push yourself through your fatigue without too much difficulty, and that you usually feel better for making the effort instead of giving in to the fatigue.

Sleepiness. This is quite different from physical fatigue, and the distinction is important. You don't feel especially tired during regular activities, but as soon as you sit on the couch, you tend to be overwhelmed by sleep. When you wake up, you're refreshed and ready to resume your day.

YOUR PERSONAL TYPE OF FATIGUE

To determine what type of fatigue you're experiencing, record your responses and refer to the chart on the opposite page.

1. Simple tiredness, with no other symptoms, is improved by resting for an hour or two. Yes ____ No ____
2. Sleepiness is the main problem, but it is improved by a short nap, with little fatigue at other times. Yes ____ No ____
3. You are apathetic, bored and always tired, but taking a short walk or performing some other activity improves your condition. Yes ____ No ____
4. You feel sick and exhausted all the time, no matter how much rest you've had, and you feel even worse after a short walk or other activity. Yes ____ No ____

Apathy and boredom. Nothing seems worth the effort when you suffer from overpowering and long-lasting fatigue. You can't think of a good reason to do anything. You can walk—you can even work—but you just don't feel like it. It's not that you're lazy; there's simply no motivation!

Sick fatigue. You are physically ill. It's as though you have the flu. Your exhaustion is accompanied by sore muscles and maybe a headache, backache or sore throat. Doing any sort of work, even mild exercise, only makes you feel worse.

HOW MUCH FATIGUE CAN YOU LIVE WITH?

Just as some people have a high tolerance of pain, some have a high tolerance of fatigue. They can go about their daily business no matter how bushed they feel. They may not like what they're doing, and they might not be doing it very well, but they do carry on.

Such people, however, are relatively rare. For most of us, the degree of fatigue we feel determines how much we can do. What is your fatigue level? What does it permit you to do in terms of daily activity?

Your Personal Fatigue Reference Chart

Use the following chart to pinpoint possible causes of fatigue.

DEGREE	TYPE	LIMITATION	MOST LIKELY CAUSE
Mild	Simple	None	Emotions, medical problem
Moderate	Simple	None to 10%	Emotions, sleep disorder, poor nutrition
Severe	Simple	10% to 50%	Emotions, medical problem
Mild	Sleepy	None	Sleep disorder
Moderate	Sleepy	10% to 25%	Sleep disorder
Severe	Sleepy	25% to 50% or more	Sleep disorder, medical problem
Mild	Apathy	None	Emotions, nutrition
Moderate	Apathy	10% to 15%	Emotions, nutrition, medical problem
Severe	Apathy	10% to 50%	Mild CFIDS, emotions
Mild	Sick	None to 10%	Emotions, medical problem
Moderate	Sick	10% to 50%	Mild CFIDS, medical problem
Severe	Sick	25% to 50% or more	CFIDS, medical problem

The following guidelines will help you realize what chronic fatigue is costing you in quality of life as well as earnings. Judge your level of fatigue on an overall average. Discount your worst and best days. Then refer to the accompanying chart to see how these parameters, combined with others, suggest likely causes of your fatigue. Note that this self-evaluation has nothing to do with other medical conditions such as joint pain, headaches and the like—just fatigue.

No limitation. You can keep going at full speed regardless of any fatigue you might feel. You don't have your usual verve or vigor, but you do get through your normal schedule.

10 percent limitation. Strenuous activities are mildly affected. You have to work harder to get the job done as well as you normally do it, but it takes no longer.

25 percent limitation. This is costing you work time. You show up late, stretch coffee breaks, add some time to your lunch hour, take afternoons off or simply skip some jobs you should do. Fatigue is definitely interfering with your activities at work and at home.

50 percent limitation. Working may be impossible for you. The few relatively good hours you have each day must be devoted to the basics of living—bathing, cooking, eating and cleaning up a bit before getting back into bed.

More than 50 percent limitation. You have to spend almost the entire day lying down. Any kind of work is out of the question. Going out for any purpose at all is impossible.

CHAPTER

5

The Tired Person's Questionnaire

Busy doctors usually get right to the point when you enter the office: "What's wrong?" they ask. Most times the answer is simple: "I broke my arm," "I have a cold" or "I can't stand these headaches."

But sometimes the answer is more complicated.

"Gee, Doc, I don't know. I feel lousy, run-down, bushed."

Unlike broken arms, colds and headaches, feeling "lousy" does not suggest a simple, by-the-book cure. The doctor has a lot more questions to ask, and you have a lot more answers to give before a diagnosis can be made and a treatment prescribed.

In chapter 4 you answered questions about the type of fatigue you feel and got a general idea about its cause. Now the following questionnaire will help you zero in on the cause. Just remember that there is often more than one factor involved, and any remedy must take all possibilities into account to be effective.

Of course, no questionnaire can replace a complete medical examination, but it can focus your thinking so you can help your physician search for the cause.

One final point: Chronic fatigue immune dysfunction syndrome (CFIDS) is sometimes a conglomeration of several individual causes. For example, if your symptoms resemble the fatigue caused by both a medical illness and a sleep disorder, and you also suffer from both anxiety and depression, think CFIDS.

As you consider the questions in this chapter, you might think that symptoms for all types of fatigue come under CFIDS. They can and sometimes do. But keep this in mind: Even though all cases of CFIDS can be classified as chronic fatigue, not all cases of chronic fatigue can be classified as CFIDS.

TIRED BECAUSE YOU'RE SICK?

These questions are basically the same ones your doctor would probably ask if you consulted him or her about your lack of energy. They deal with the general characteristics of medical illnesses and some of the easily diagnosed conditions that may contribute to, or even be entirely responsible for, your fatigue.

Have you ever been diagnosed with any serious medical condition? If the answer is yes, maybe you have it again, and that may be causing or contributing to your fatigue. Some people, for example, have repeated episodes of fatigue-inducing anemia. Other illnesses, such as arthritis or thyroid disease, can also lead to bouts of fatigue. A physical examination and laboratory tests will reveal these simple causes.

Do you have any current medical illnesses? Maybe your doctor is treating you for an ailment and neglected to tell you that fatigue is one of the side effects of the condition. Ask your doctor if this is so in your case.

Of course, the very nature of any illness can lead to fatigue. After all, the body uses up a lot of energy in fighting disease and recovering from it.

Is your illness under medical control? Many illnesses, such as diabetes or chronic infections, can cause deep fatigue if they are poorly treated or out of control. Proper medical attention may improve energy levels substantially and eliminate fatigue completely.

Do you take any prescription medications? Many prescription and nonprescription drugs have fatigue as a side effect. Among the most common of these are blood pressure medications, antihistamines, pain medications and tranquilizers or antidepressants. If you are taking any regular medication, ask your physician if it can cause fatigue and if there's a less tiring alternative.

Here is a quick look at some common medical conditions that are often likened to fatigue, plus some basic questions that could tell you if you do have such a condition.

If your answer to any of these questions is yes, you might want to see your doctor.

Chronic Anemia

1. Are you uncharacteristically pale? Yes ____ No ____
2. Are you exhausted by simple exertion such as walking up stairs but feel fine while resting? Yes ____ No ____
3. Do you get short of breath easily? Yes ____ No ____
4. Does your heart pound during any exertion? Yes ____ No ____
5. Does your heart race during any exertion? Yes ____ No ____
6. Do you have excessive blood loss, such as a heavy menstrual flow? Yes ____ No ____

If you have anemia, that means that you have too few red cells in the bloodstream to carry enough oxygen to the tissues. Its causes range from simple nutritional deficiency to genetic predisposition.

But don't blame anemia for your fatigue if your blood count (the number of red cells in your bloodstream) is borderline. If you suffer from bone-crushing exhaustion and only mild anemia, the cause of your fatigue is probably something else. On the other hand, some people with severe anemia feel relatively well, particularly when resting.

Diabetes Mellitus

1. Do you urinate frequently? Yes ____ No ____
2. Are you overweight? Yes ____ No ____
3. Do you crave sweets? Yes ____ No ____
4. Is there a history of diabetes in your family? Yes ____ No ____
5. Are cuts and sores slow to heal? Yes ____ No ____

Diabetes mellitus, sometimes known as sugar diabetes, is extremely common. But as millions of diabetics know, it can be treated effectively with diet and, if necessary, oral medications or insulin injections. Diabetes is an easy disease to spot during a routine medical exam.

Hypothyroidism

1. Do you have excessive hair loss? Yes ____ No ____
2. Is your hair thicker than before? Yes ____ No ____
3. Does cold weather bother you considerably?
Yes ____ No ____
4. Do you have swelling in the front of your neck?
Yes ____ No ____
5. Are you chronically constipated? Yes ____ No ____

The thyroid hormone, thyroxine, is essential to a sense of well-being and vitality. An underactive thyroid (hypothyroidism) is a common condition, but it usually comes on so gradually that it may be hard to tie it to the onset of the fatigue. Simple blood tests or a complete physical examination will readily identify this condition.

Arthritis

1. Do your joints hurt? Yes ____ No ____
2. Are your joints swollen? Yes ____ No ____
3. When you wake up in the morning, are your joints stiff? Yes ____ No ____
4. Is there a history of arthritis in your family?
Yes ____ No ____
5. Do you have blood in your urine? Yes ____ No ____

The word *arthritis* does not denote a single disease. It is a general term for many different types of joint problems. One of the more worrisome ones is lupus erythematosus, and if you answer yes to the last question in this group, you should be checked specifically for this condition.

Chronic Infections

1. Do you have infections that do not heal? Yes ____ No ____
2. Is tonsillitis a common problem for you? Yes ____ No ____
3. Do you suffer from ongoing sinus infections?
Yes ____ No ____
4. Do you have urinary tract infections frequently?
Yes ____ No ____

5. Is there a history of frequent infections in your family? Yes ____ No ____

Frequent or long-standing infections are seldom the main cause of chronic fatigue. Still, some people simply ignore persistent infections because they don't want to spend money to see a doctor or they're afraid of what they might discover. Sometimes they simply refuse to accept the fact that something is wrong with them. They are determined to live with the problem as long as they can stand it. If you suffer from chronic or long-standing infections, taking care of them just might ease your fatigue.

Multiple Allergies

1. Do you have common allergies—pollen, foods, dogs, certain fabrics and such? Yes ____ No ____
2. Is your fatigue worse when your allergies act up? Yes ____ No ____
3. Do you have asthma? Yes ____ No ____
4. Do you feel worse in certain environments? Yes ____ No ____
5. Is there a history of allergies in your family? Yes ____ No ____
6. Do you take antihistamines to treat your allergies? Yes ____ No ____
7. Are you unable to tolerate certain foods (milk or wheat, for example)? Yes ____ No ____

People can be allergic to a whole range of substances, but those with allergies accompanied by fatigue are usually able to tie the two together. During hay-fever season, for example, they sneeze and sniffle because of ragweed pollen, and as their allergy symptoms get worse, their fatigue increases. In the winter, when ragweed pollen is gone, they don't feel tired. The connection is clear.

Food allergies may not be so obvious, especially if they involve additives or other ingredients we consume without even knowing it. You might be totally unaware that the reason you feel so poorly is that there was monosodium glutamate (MSG) in the sweet-and-sour pork you ate last night. And if you can't make that connection, you might not link your fatigue with MSG, either.

Lyme Disease

1. Were you ever bitten by a tick? Yes ____ No ____

2. Did you have an unusual, persistent rash around the site of the tick bite? Yes ____ No ____
3. Did you develop joint pain after the tick bite? Yes ____ No ____
4. Do you hike in the fields or woods as a sport or hobby or as part of your job? Yes ____ No ____

The deer tick, which carries the Lyme disease infection, is particularly common in Connecticut, New York and Massachusetts, but it shows up in many other parts of the United States as well. Lyme disease causes fatigue as a side effect, and it can be difficult to diagnose. However, there are specific blood tests for the disease, and if you suspect that you have it, tell your doctor to include that test as part of your complete physical examination.

AIDS (HIV Infection)

1. Did you have a blood transfusion between 1980 and 1983? Yes ____ No ____
2. Have you used recreational drugs intravenously? Yes ____ No ____
3. Are you gay or bisexual, and do you practice unprotected sex? Yes ____ No ____
4. Have you or your partner ever had unprotected sex? Yes ____ No ____

Fatigue, along with chronic infections and other manifestations of damage to the immune system, is a prominent symptom of AIDS. Many who suffer from chronic fatigue worry that it might be due to AIDS, even though they have no risk factors.

If you have any doubts at all, have the HIV test. It is easy, accurate and inexpensive (perhaps even free in your state), and it provides much peace of mind.

Cancer

1. Do you have unusual lumps or swelling? Yes ____ No ____
2. Have you noticed any unusual bleeding? Yes ____ No ____
3. Do you bruise easily? Yes ____ No ____
4. Are you losing significant weight without dieting? Yes ____ No ____
5. Is there a history of cancer in your family? Yes ____ No ____

Fatigue can be a prominent symptom of cancer in its early stages. But this disease provokes so much fear that millions of people would rather not know if they have it. Instead of consulting a doctor about their fatigue and the possibility that it might be a sign of cancer, some people refuse to mention their suspicion—and worry about it constantly instead. The worry just increases their fatigue and gives any cancer present more time to spread.

Mention any concerns about cancer to your doctor. If you have been plagued by fatigue for more than a year and a complete physical examination does not reveal any malignancy, take a deep breath and relax. You'll have to look elsewhere for the cause. However, like everyone else, you should continue to have regular cancer checkups. Even if tests reveal a malignancy, there's hope. Cancer can be cured, particularly when it is caught early.

Sleep Disorders

1. Do you have insomnia? Yes ____ No ____
2. Is it difficult for you to get to sleep? Yes ____ No ____
3. Do you take pills to help you fall asleep? Yes ____ No ____
4. Do you wake frequently during the night? Yes ____ No ____
5. During sleep, do you experience muscle jerking or twitching? Yes ____ No ____
6. Do you snore loudly? Yes ____ No ____
7. When you wake in the morning, do you feel unrefreshed? Yes ____ No ____
8. Do you wake with a headache? Yes ____ No ____

It's obvious that without a good night's sleep, you can't expect to have much energy or vitality the next day. When a whole month goes by and you haven't had a good night's sleep, you'll probably find yourself lurching like a zombie.

Strange as it may seem, physicians are only now becoming aware of just how important sleep is to overall health and how sleep disorders complicate other medical problems.

Loss of sleep also contributes to many of the specific fatigue syndromes like jet lag and shift worker's fatigue, and these circumstances complicate many medical causes of fatigue. If, for example, you're in pain because you broke your arm, hurt your back or your arthritis is acting up, you probably won't sleep very well.

Sleep disorders, like stress and depression, are rarely the sole cause of chronic fatigue, but they can be a complicating factor.

Nutritional Deficiency

1. Do you pay little attention to your diet? Yes ____ No ____
2. Are you overweight? Yes ____ No ____
3. Do you crave sweets? Yes ____ No ____
4. Do you eat sweets to get a lift? Yes ____ No ____
5. Do you have a weakness for candy, snacks or other junk food? Yes ____ No ____
6. Do you avoid eating dairy products, vegetables or any other major food group? Yes ____ No ____
7. Are you negligent about getting calorie-burning exercise? Yes ____ No ____

If you fill your body with low-energy foods, you can expect a low-energy performance. How can you expect to feel any sense of vitality if your diet, the source of your energy, consists of junk food?

And getting a quick sugar-based energy fix isn't the solution, either. A nutritious and well-balanced diet is essential for sustained energy levels as well as a healthy weight level and a sense of well-being.

Stress

1. Do you consider yourself a nervous person? Yes ____ No ____
2. Are you unable to sit and relax? Yes ____ No ____
3. Are you too sensitive to criticism? Yes ____ No ____
4. Do you feel that tremendous pressures are placed on you? Yes ____ No ____
5. Do you find it hard to relax away from work? Yes ____ No ____
6. Do you drink more than five cups of coffee a day? Yes ____ No ____
7. Do you feel you have to solve everyone else's problems? Yes ____ No ____
8. Have you any unrealistic fears? Yes ____ No ____
9. Do you drink alcohol to relax? Yes ____ No ____
10. Are you on tranquilizing drugs? Yes ____ No ____
11. Do you have trouble gaining weight? Yes ____ No ____
12. Is it hard for you to get to sleep? Yes ____ No ____

13. Are you obsessed with personal health matters?
Yes ____ No ____

Being nervous takes a lot out of you: constant tension; jumping at sounds; flying off the handle at the slightest annoyance; nervous tics, twitches and habits; and all the other physical manifestations of stress require a great deal of energy. And that energy, once used, is no longer available to help you handle other areas of your life.

Although chronic stress inevitably leads to fatigue, it is not always the sole cause. Many people are stressed by medical disorders and conditions that complicate and intensify their fatigue.

Depression

1. Are you depressed? Yes ____ No ____
2. Do you feel discouraged? Yes ____ No ____
3. Are you unhappy with the way your life is going?
Yes ____ No ____
4. Are you unable to communicate with friends or family? Yes ____ No ____
5. Have you considered suicide? Yes ____ No ____
6. Do you have a history of emotional disorders?
Yes ____ No ____
7. Do all activities seem boring? Yes ____ No ____

Depression, like stress, robs you of energy. Even worse, it can make your lack of energy seem unimportant. As with stress, depression is not always the main cause of fatigue, but it can complicate and aggravate the situation.

CFIDS

At the beginning of this chapter, we stated that CFIDS can be seen as a combination of all the causes of fatigue. If you answered yes to half of the symptoms under anemia, hypothyroidism, arthritis and allergy, it's likely that you have CFIDS.

While it is a medical condition, most of those who have CFIDS also suffer from sleep disorders and depression. Stress clearly aggravates CFIDS.

If you answer yes to the majority of the following questions, CFIDS is probably the cause of your fatigue. The diagnosis of

CFIDS overrides all the other individual causes, such as sleep disorder, stress and depression.

1. Are you functioning at less than half of your usual pace? Yes ____ No ____
2. Have you been feeling tired for at least six months? Yes ____ No ____
3. Does your tiredness seem to be a "sick" exhaustion? Yes ____ No ____
4. Does exertion make the fatigue worse? Yes ____ No ____
5. Do you feel as though you have the flu all the time? Yes ____ No ____
6. Do you have chronic headaches? Yes ____ No ____
7. Do you have frequent sore throats? Yes ____ No ____
8. Do your lymph glands swell and hurt? Yes ____ No ____
9. Is it hard for you to remember or concentrate? Yes ____ No ____
10. Are your joints painful? Yes ____ No ____
11. Are your muscles sore? Yes ____ No ____
12. Do your eyes ache? Yes ____ No ____
13. Are your eyes sensitive to light? Yes ____ No ____
14. Do you have stomach pains, diarrhea and/or constipation? Yes ____ No ____
15. Do your arms or legs feel numb or weak? Yes ____ No ____
16. Do you sleep poorly and wake unrefreshed? Yes ____ No ____
17. Do you feel as though you have a fever but show no temperature elevation? Yes ____ No ____
18. Do you get chills? Yes ____ No ____
19. Do you have night sweats? Yes ____ No ____
20. Do your cheeks flush? Yes ____ No ____
21. Do you need to urinate frequently? Yes ____ No ____
22. Are you depressed? Yes ____ No ____
23. Does stress worsen your symptoms? Yes ____ No ____
24. Do you have allergies? Yes ____ No ____

Patients with CFIDS will have answered yes to at least 15 of these questions. Some who are very ill with CFIDS answer yes to all of them. Even so, most physicians are reluctant to make the diagnosis of this common and devastating medical problem.

WHAT DO I DO NOW?

Study the results of this questionnaire, plus the chart you filled out in the last chapter. Think about your answers and what they reveal about your life, the way you feel and how you think about yourself. Do this for a day or so, then ask yourself the following questions.

1. Do I still agree with the answers I wrote down?
2. Are they an honest assessment of myself, my ailments and the possible causes of my condition?
3. Is there any pattern?
4. Do I see anything I can do right now, any changes I can make in the way I live, work and play, that could change my life in a positive way?
5. Am I ready to work toward the long-term goal of ending or at least easing the chronic fatigue that is destroying my life?

You might want to wait a few more days, then once again answer the questions from this chapter and chapter 4 on a separate sheet of paper. Compare the answers. If some of the answers don't match, try to figure out why, and if you can't decide, make a note of the differences.

When you've finished the questionnaires, studied your answers and done some reading to familiarize yourself with the various problems that might be causing or contributing to your fatigue, you're ready for the next step—a long visit with your doctor.

CHAPTER 6

When to See Your Doctor

If you're unlucky enough to come down with a bad cold or a case of the flu, you know you'll be miserable for a few days, then it will probably pass and you'll be back to normal in a week or so. But if your condition turns nasty—the sniffles never stop or the chest congestion becomes a battle for breath—you call a doctor for professional help.

When you're sidelined by a spell of sheer exhaustion, you slow down and get some rest. Certainly the tiredness will disappear in a few hours or a few days, and you'll regain your energy. But if the fatigue persists for weeks or months and takes over your life, you must see a physician.

Don't try to deal with chronic fatigue by yourself. Success is unlikely, and even more serious health problems could result. Excessive tiredness is a medical condition. That's why any treatment program must start with a visit to your doctor to determine if some physical or medical condition is aggravating the problem or interfering with treatment.

Not all fatigue-causing conditions fit neatly into the "medical" category. For example, neither dieting nor exercising is a medical condition, but each can have medical consequences. Pregnancy is neither a disease nor an illness, but it is definitely a physical condition that can cause or contribute to fatigue. So can nursing a baby.

Even if your lack of energy is primarily due to stress or depression, it's likely that some other medical factors either aggravate or complicate it. Don't cheat yourself out of a complete recovery by second-guessing the need for a physical exam.

Quite often, tracing the origins of your fatigue is like peeling an onion. You uncover the first layer, check it for clues, then go on to the next layer. This produces a lot of negative information. That is, you learn what is *not* causing the fatigue—also very important information. For example, if your doctor finds that you don't have cancer, simple anemia, diabetes mellitus or hypothyroidism, they are eliminated as the cause of your constant fatigue. The more possibilities you can eliminate, the closer you are to the real cause.

But this kind of detective work takes patience, both on your part and the part of your doctor. That's why you should be forewarned before your first appointment to get to the root of your perpetual tiredness.

WHY DOCTORS OFTEN DODGE FATIGUE COMPLAINTS

Don't be surprised if the response is cool when you tell the doctor your problem is chronic fatigue. Generally speaking, doctors are reluctant to deal with it. Here's why.

Physicians would rather not spend extended periods with individual patients. Their waiting rooms are crowded, and they try to see everybody. If the visits are short, patients don't get backed up in the waiting room. But no simple test can spot, let alone measure, the extent of chronic fatigue. That means repetitive testing and long-term observation are necessary for proper diagnosis. Also, technology fails physicians miserably when they deal with a problem of this type.

Let's see how these reasons govern the manner in which some doctors treat a potential case of chronic fatigue.

A patient comes in with a basic complaint about being tired all the time. During the interview the patient happens to mention having a sore throat. The doctor is likely to concentrate completely on the sore throat.

From a doctor's point of view, sore throats are a piece of cake. They're easy to examine, easy to diagnose and easy to treat. Best of all, regardless of what treatment the doctor prescribes, a sore throat is almost sure to go away.

Any mention of fatigue is blamed on the throat infection. The fatigue will disappear, says the doctor, when the sore throat does. Obviously there is no need for an entire battery of tests, which are both time-consuming and costly.

After a throat culture is done and a little penicillin is prescribed, the patient is out the door. The patient's fatigue complaint was barely even acknowledged!

TEN WAYS TO HELP YOUR DOCTOR TREAT FATIGUE

When you consult a doctor about persistent fatigue, you have to remember that few physicians know very much about the problem. (This is changing, but slowly.) In fact, if you want your doctor to make a serious attempt at finding the cause and helping you recover, it might be necessary for you to take part in your doctor's education. Here's how to do it.

1. Since the subject of fatigue cannot be dealt with adequately in the average ten-minute visit, make an appointment for a complete medical exam.
2. Let the doctor, or at least the receptionist, know that the reason you want a complete examination is because you feel tired—excessively tired—most or all of the time. Make sure enough time is scheduled for you to describe and discuss your symptoms.
3. When talking to the doctor, keep the focus of the discussion on your lack of energy. Don't allow yourself or the physician to get sidetracked by other issues. Using the questionnaires in chapters 4 and 5, make notes before your visit to make sure you cover all the points that concern you.
4. Know your subject. But don't imply that you know more than your doctor—even if it appears that you really do. After all, you are there for the doctor's medical opinion, so make sure you get it.
5. Know your symptoms. Be as concrete and specific as possible. If you say you need more sleep, say how much sleep you get now. If you tried something that didn't work, tell the doctor exactly what you did.

6. Talk honestly about any emotional or psychological issues you are dealing with: problems with a relationship, depression, a family member's drinking or drug use, your own chemical dependency, the loss of a loved one, being out of work—anything that could be a contributing factor. It could be that your problem is psychological or emotional and not physical at all.
7. Don't argue with your doctor. This will only cause resentment, and it might result in your getting less than the compassionate care you deserve. Patients who go in with the attitude that they already know it all just waste their money and their doctor's time.
8. Realize that physicians and medical science have their limitations.
9. If your doctor knows little about chronic fatigue but is open to investigating it and finding out more about what you are going through, give him a copy of this book.
10. If all else fails, look for another doctor—one who will take you and your problems seriously; one who practices the art of medicine as well as the technology.

Most doctors say that they enjoy treating a knowledgeable patient who sincerely wants an opinion. They take it as a compliment when patients have read up on their symptoms and really want to know what the doctor thinks.

WHAT TO EXPECT IN A COMPLETE PHYSICAL EXAM

When you sign up for a complete physical, you should get a head-to-toe examination, including the full cancer screening recommended by the American Cancer Society. In the process, the doctor will do a lot of poking and prodding and ask you a lot of questions to see what, if anything, is abnormal about you.

Is the size of your liver and your lymph nodes normal? Do you have any breast lumps? Are the results of the pelvic and rectal exams normal? Is the prostate gland enlarged? Is there any minor swelling of the joint tissue in your wrists? The physician will ask you if your hair is thickening or falling out and will check the skin texture of your hands, which might suggest certain types of disease.

You don't have to understand the technical aspects of the exam. You can tell by your own good sense if you received a superficial once-over or a careful study. Don't settle for anything less than a thorough examination, if that's what you requested.

These tests should be performed routinely on persons who suspect a chronic fatigue problem:

- Complete blood count to check for anemia and chronic infections.
- Sedimentation rate test. It is a simple, inexpensive and useful way to screen a variety of medical abnormalities that suggest further investigation.
- Routine chemistries. Thyroid and arthritis tests are essential to rule out many of the medical illnesses that cause fatigue.
- Chest x-ray. This should be mandatory for all persons with unexplained fatigue.

If these results are normal, prominent symptoms may indicate the need for further detailed laboratory testing. That's when you need to know your physician can be trusted to follow all leads with appropriate and cost-effective testing. You want a thorough exam, not an excessive one.

Always feel free to ask your doctor what tests are being done and why. If you don't understand the first explanation, ask for a simpler one. Doctors know how to speak in simple English, but sometimes they have to be reminded to do it.

If your physician does diagnose the cause of your lost energy, pay close attention to treatment suggestions. They should involve more than just a prescription for some medicine. Ask questions that will help you explore other ways to deal with tiredness and fatigue. If no diagnosis is made, stay in touch with your doctor. You will still need ongoing care and periodic evaluation, and you will want to be informed of any new developments in the testing or treatment of chronic fatigue.

Think of your physician as a friend who will explore personal matters with you. If you couple the informational resources available to you with advice from your physician, you will contribute significantly to solving the puzzle of your tiredness. Always remember that chronic fatigue is a medical condition, and the search for a solution starts at your doctor's office.

PART II
WINNING STRATEGIES AGAINST FATIGUE

CHAPTER 7

Solutions to Medically Based Fatigue

It takes a lot of energy to be sick. And that energy is stolen from the rest of your life. You know only too well that being sick usually makes you too tired to do much of anything.

While the body is fighting off an attack from a viral infection or an allergen, all of its available strength is thrown at the attacker. So while that critical battle is being waged, the rest of our mind and body just drones along, content to keep operating at minimal efficiency.

In some cases we're lucky if we can do even that. Some medical conditions can cause profound and disabling fatigue, so that we are both achy *and* tired, or burning up with fever *and* tired, or in pain *and* tired.

Sometimes that tiredness turns out to be a plus. Let's say, for example, that you have a three-day viral infection, complete with muscle aches, headache, backache, sinus pain, sore throat and hacking cough. Your fatigue forces you to rest and sleep, giving your body a chance to fight the virus and renew itself, while you sleep through some of the discomfort.

But chronic, inexplicable fatigue can be a subtle hint of an underlying—but very treatable—medical condition. Let's first consider diet and digestive problems.

DISORDERED DIGESTION

If the cycle that turns food into energy is disrupted, you lose out on that energy. And when the disruption is serious and lasting, the loss becomes disabling, if not life-threatening.

One obvious sign of such a problem is severe weight loss. If you crash diet or exercise too strenuously while eating too few calories, the body uses up its fat reserves, then begins to burn up energy reserves stored in muscle mass. The faster the condition develops, the greater the degree of fatigue.

But even though we live in a society that encourages dieting for weight control and slimness, weight loss is not always desirable. This is certainly true when the weight loss is due to physical illness or compulsive or obsessive behavior such as anorexia nervosa and bulimia.

Anorexia nervosa. Some people literally starve themselves. For reasons often tied in with a poor self-image and other emotional problems, anorexics—most commonly adolescent girls and young women—are convinced that they have to lose weight, no matter what the bathroom scale might say. They may be 10, 20, 30 or more pounds underweight but feel that they are too fat. For them it's always losing just a few more pounds that will make things right. They don't want to eat. Even the thought of eating can make them physically ill.

Like alcoholics, drug addicts and other victims of self-destructive or obsessive behavior, anorexics often deny that they have a problem. If forced to confront their dangerous behavior pattern, they may lie about their willingness to seek help; they take the food, then hide it or throw it away. Without outside help, they might starve themselves to death.

Because theirs is a psychological as well as medical condition, it is crucial that anorexics get professional care. Various treatment programs and self-help groups address this problem. If you think you or someone you love suffers from anorexia, seek help immediately.

Bulimia. Like anorexics, bulimics have problems with self-image and self-worth and are terrified of being what they consider fat. But unlike anorexics, bulimics *do* eat. In fact, they often gorge themselves. They eat for the sake of eating. They are compulsive, like alcoholics and drug addicts.

Some people are both anorexic and bulimic. They starve themselves for a time and then go on to an eating binge. Immediately following the binge, they deliberately vomit or take laxatives or diuretics as a way to avoid gaining weight. The food is expelled or eliminated before it can be digested and used to produce energy. This is called a binge-and-purge cycle. These people risk developing a wide range of serious and long-lasting physical problems on top of the psychological problems that caused their bulimia.

Lack of energy is the least of their problems. Like anorexia, bulimia is a life-threatening psychological as well as physical illness. Those afflicted with it are urged to enroll in a treatment program that helps address both issues.

Malabsorption syndromes. When the intestines are obstructed or even partially blocked, vomiting, fatigue and weight loss will occur even in someone who is eating well. Some people suffer from malabsorption syndromes that prevent the food from being absorbed through the lining of the intestine. Also, bowel disorders, such as Crohn's disease or colitis, cause diarrhea and decreased food absorption, all of which lead to fatigue. These conditions are usually easy to diagnose and treat.

Obesity. Like a car, the human body uses gas (energy) even when it's idling. And in the same way a limousine uses more energy while idling than a compact car, an obese person uses more energy at rest than a thinner person does. When the action starts, then energy consumption climbs.

But that's only one reason obese people are prone to chronic fatigue. Their bodies also do not produce energy efficiently enough to handle that extra weight. And obese people usually have nutritional problems.

In cases of extreme obesity the problems increase, preventing victims from breathing properly. That translates into less oxygen for the bloodstream, meaning reduced energy production, which compounds the problem.

Extreme obesity can lead to more than chronic fatigue. All in all, obesity is associated with 50 medical conditions, some of them life-threatening.

Diet is the basic treatment for fatigue due to obesity, but don't depend on one of those quickie diets you read about in supermarket tabloids. It takes time to gain a lot of weight, and it takes time to lose it, too. Consult your doctor about the best weight-loss plan for you. Any cut in intake is likely to cause some fatigue at first, but it's only temporary.

We'll look at obesity as a cause of fatigue in greater detail in chapter 14. Many health experts consider obesity the number one health problem in America today.

COMMON CONDITIONS THAT SAP YOUR ENERGY

There are a number of other surprising—but all too commonplace—causes of fatigue among adults.

Heart disease. Once oxygen is absorbed into the bloodstream, it must still be transported to the tissues so it can combine with glucose to produce energy. It takes a lot of power to pump blood through the bloodstream. A weak heart can't do that efficiently, and without the necessary pumping power, poor tissue oxygenation may result.

But even a strong heart cannot unblock clogged arteries. Good circulation also requires wide-open arteries. And what is one of the main symptoms of either clogged arteries or a weak heart? Fatigue.

If you do suffer from heart or circulatory problems, your doctor should be able to spot it. If you're feeling unusually tired for no apparent reason and you come from a family with a history of heart disease, a cholesterol test might be a good idea.

Arthritis. This chronic inflammation of the joint tissue raises the energy needs of the body. That's why chronic fatigue is a prominent symptom in certain types of arthritis, notably rheumatoid arthritis and lupus erythematosus. However, like most fatigue-related medical conditions, tiredness is not the number one symptom of arthritis. It is usually third or fourth on the list.

One increasingly common form of arthritis is Lyme disease, caused by a bacteria transmitted in tick bites. The fatigue is induced by the body's increased energy requirements as it tries to fight a chronic infection plus chronic inflammation. Even though the fatigue due to Lyme disease can be very severe, it usually diminishes when accurately diagnosed and treated. If you spend any amount of time in the woods, check yourself for a red rash that resembles a bull's-eye, and get treatment promptly if you suspect you've been bitten.

Diabetes mellitus. Usually linked to advancing age and obesity, this type of fatigue-causing diabetes may not be easily recognized because the symptoms appear and worsen very gradually. Eventually those with diabetes think of their constant fatigue, thirst and frequent urination as "normal."

Their fatigue, while generalized and pervasive, is relatively subtle and may not even be mentioned during a visit to the doctor. After all, many older or obese people expect to be more tired than their younger and slimmer friends. Later, when the diabetes is treated and is under control, the victims notice a dramatic improvement in energy levels.

Routine blood and urine tests readily identify the presence of diabetes, since its primary characteristic is an excess of glucose in the bloodstream, due to a shortage of the hormone insulin. Without insulin, glucose is not absorbed by the body's cells: No glucose, no energy. Fortunately, diabetes is relatively easy to control. It requires weight loss, careful dietary measures and, in some cases, medication or insulin. Once the diabetes is under control, the fatigue disappears and the person usually feels youthfully energetic again.

Hypothyroidism. Let's examine the thyroid gland itself in preparation for considering hypothyroidism. It is a butterfly-shaped organ located in the front of the neck. The gland produces thyroxine, a hormone that is directly involved in regulating the body's metabolism. That is what determines how well and how fast you use the energy you produce.

If the gland is underactive, it won't produce enough thyroxine, and the machine you know as your body will slow down. You'll have hypothyroidism, and fatigue will ensue.

Of all the illness-related causes of chronic fatigue, hypothyroidism is probably the most insidious. The fatigue creeps up gradually, sapping the strength and energy needed for daily activities.

Other symptoms include thickened hair, dulled emotions and a sensitivity to cold weather. The lower metabolic rate can also produce a lower body temperature.

Anyone who suffers from chronic fatigue should be tested for hypothyroidism. If thyroxine is low, administering the hormone will almost always restore lost energy.

Hyperthyroidism. As you probably suspect, this is the opposite of hypothyroidism: With hyperthyroidism your thyroid is overactive and your metabolism runs too fast, burning energy like a car gunning its engine while stuck in traffic. It gulps fuel and doesn't go anywhere. This waste can cause weight loss, an intolerance of hot weather, diarrhea, nervousness—and fatigue.

The same blood tests used to detect hypothyroidism can also identify hyperthyroidism.

Breathing disorders. It takes oxygen to convert the food you eat to energy. But any problem or disruption in the respiratory cycle can limit the amount of oxygen that reaches the bloodstream. The result—fatigue.

In respiratory disorders such as chronic bronchitis or emphysema, the lungs' air sacs don't work properly. Too little oxygen is absorbed into the bloodstream, resulting in reduced energy production.

In the early stages, lung disease may cause problems only during exertion. But, as the condition worsens, any activity might lead to shortness of breath or chest pains. Any breathing problems should be reported to your physician, whether or not you're low on energy. Fortunately, lung disease of all kinds—from common ailments to rare problems like asbestos contamination or birth defects—are relatively easy to diagnose.

Anemia. Red blood cells carry the iron- and oxygen-rich molecules called hemoglobin to tissues throughout the body. Any decrease in the number of red blood cells, called anemia, means less oxygen reaches the tissues. As with heart disease, a shortage of oxygen in the blood cells results in fatigue.

Anemia is one of the few conditions where fatigue may be the only symptom you have.

A complete blood count (CBC) will pinpoint anemia. It's a simple laboratory test that anyone who experiences regular bouts of fatigue should have done. Unfortunately, what keeps many people from seeking—and getting—relief is that they can and do adjust to being anemic. For many people with the condition, the fatigue is relatively mild, noticeable only after exercise and exertion. In more severe cases, the fatigue can be profound.

Fatigue is most noticeable when anemia develops quickly. People who are used to high loads of oxygen in their bloodstream feel the drop more acutely than those who are accustomed to reduced levels. Surprisingly, some people with chronic anemia are barely aware of their fatigue. They adapt to it and arrange their lives so that they can take advantage of whatever energy they do have.

Among the many causes of anemia, the most common is iron deficiency resulting from poor dietary habits or excessive loss of blood, such as in heavy menstrual flow. Other causes range from impaired hemoglobin production in the blood cells to increased rates of red blood cell breakdown. If you are anemic, your physician should be able to tell you the exact cause and the best way to improve or correct it.

For more on nutritional deficiencies as a cause of fatigue, see chapter 14, which covers the topic in more detail.

IMMUNE PROBLEMS THAT CAN LEAVE YOU LISTLESS

When your immune system goes on the offensive, battling internal and external enemies, something's got to give. And usually that "something" is your stamina.

Allergies and allergy medication. Multiple allergies cause a nagging fatigue that compounds all the other symptoms: sneezing, coughing, itchy eyes and runny nose.

Allergies are a result of our immune system's attempt to protect us from foreign substances. Sometimes it overreacts and fights against harmless substances such as pollen or dust. It takes a lot of energy to keep the sneezing, coughing, itchy eyes and runny nose going all day. This leads to fatigue. When we take medication, we hope to end the symptoms and the accompanying fatigue; ironically, the antihistamine medication most commonly used to treat allergies has fatigue as a major side effect. But that is a different kind of fatigue—drug-based fatigue, which we'll discuss later in this chapter.

Fortunately, newer medications can ease some allergies without making you drowsy or listless. Ask your allergy doctor about them.

Chronic infection. Infections are a part of life. That's why you have an immune system that helps you cope with bacteria, viruses, toxins and so forth. Sometimes, however, an infection becomes so firmly established that the body can't shake it off. This is usually due to some other problem, stress or some other factor that's compromising your immune system.

Let's look at a chronic sinus infection as an example. The sinuses may be blocked because of an allergy, multiple allergies or smoking. Any or all of them can help turn a one-time sinus infection into a chronic problem.

Once a chronic infection is established, it takes a lot of body energy to fight it. That energy is diverted from other uses, such as working, playing, pursuing projects and enjoying friends and family.

Some chronic infections drain more energy than others. In fact, some demand more energy than your body can produce. You and your doctor, working together, can make up the deficit through diet and medication.

Tuberculosis (TB) is a good example. Chronic TB causes fatigue—among other symptoms—because of the oxygen-depriving lung disease it produces and because of the increased energy it demands. Ongoing or chronic urinary tract infections, yeast and other fungal infections or a mysterious fever can also sap energy. All of these can be detected by your doctor. So don't suffer in silence—check in for a checkup.

AIDS (acquired immune deficiency syndrome). Severe fatigue is one of the earliest symptoms of AIDS. In the first stages, the fatigue is caused by an overactive immune system fighting the virus. In the later stages, this fatigue is compounded by the numerous chronic infections that overcome the weakened immune system, take hold and eventually kill the AIDS victim.

AIDS is caused by the human immunodeficiency virus (HIV) and spreads through contact with infected blood and other body fluids. Therefore, getting a transfusion with HIV-infected blood, sharing contaminated hypodermic needles during drug use and having sexual intercourse with an infected person can all cause the disease. This isn't meant to scare you—if you're not in a high-risk category, there's no need to lie awake nights terrified that you have AIDS; you'll just get more and more tired due to lack of rest. If you're worried, however, it would be worth your peace of mind to get tested for HIV. Although there is no cure now, AIDS can be diagnosed readily and treated symptomatically.

Mononucleosis and the Epstein-Barr virus. At one point many researchers believed that the Epstein-Barr virus (EBV) caused chronic fatigue immune dysfunction syndrome (CFIDS) as well as mononucleosis. Today we know it does not cause CFIDS.

But the Epstein-Barr virus does definitely cause mononucleosis, or mono, also known as the kissing disease because the virus can be found in the saliva and transmitted orally: by sharing food, eating utensils or a cup—or by kissing.

Even though 95 percent of all adults have had EBV, few of us knew it at the time because the infection was so mild that we probably passed it off as a slight touch of the flu.

Once you get EBV, you have it for life. It's part of the herpes virus family, and like all herpes viruses, it never leaves the body.

When EBV does develop into mono, it lasts for two or three weeks before resolving itself. It is sometimes referred to as glandular fever because it produces swollen glands, fever, a sore throat—and fatigue. Severe cases are called infectious mononucleosis. Its victims become seriously fatigued—possibly for months.

WHEN THE TREATMENT LEAVES YOU WEAK

Sometimes fatigue is a side effect of convalescence or medication.

Recovery or healing. Not being sick does not necessarily mean being well.

Let's say you've recovered from an ailment of some kind. Maybe you broke your leg and had it set. You're getting along with crutches, a walking cast or a cane. But it can still take days, weeks or even months for you to regain your strength—your energy.

Give yourself time to convalesce from an illness or an injury. If you push yourself before you have all your energy back, you may suffer a relapse or incur a new ailment due to weakness.

A hidden medical cause—drugs. A list of all the prescription and nonprescription drugs that can cause fatigue would fill more than 300 pages. Doctors and patients routinely overlook this simple fact. And when you add a new medication to the ones you already take, you can cook up a chemical stew with even more and worse side effects.

For this reason, it's a good idea to get all your prescriptions at one pharmacy. The pharmacist can track all of the medications you're using and spot a conflict your doctor might miss, especially if you see more than one doctor.

There are three primary ways in which drugs can cause fatigue: by decreasing energy production, by interfering with energy utilization and by increasing energy requirements. Browse through the *Physician's Desk Reference* or another guide to medications, and it is easy to see that nearly every drug has the potential to cause fatigue. It might not be the culprit in your case, but if you are taking medication and have chronic fatigue, ask your physician, your pharmacist or both if the medication could be the cause.

Blood pressure medications, for example, are notorious for causing fatigue. A nonpharmaceutical alternative such as exercising, losing weight, changing your diet, giving up smoking or drinking or reducing stress might restore your energy. If, however, your high blood pressure does require medication, ask your doctor to prescribe a drug that causes minimal or no fatigue.

If both your illness and your medication cause fatigue, talk to your doctor. The two of you should be able to come up with a solution. If your doctor approves, you may be able to taper off the medication for a while to see if your fatigue disappears. If it does, you know that the drug may have been the cause.

By the way, antibiotics generally don't apply here. They rarely cause chronic fatigue by themselves, and if they are used to treat an established infection, your energy levels should improve markedly as the drugs take effect. But heavy or frequent reliance on antibiotics might encourage yeast infections. As we saw earlier, all types of infections can cause fatigue—and chronic infections can lead to chronic fatigue.

RARE CAUSES OF FATIGUE

You're eating well, your food is being digested and stored as energy, and your body is able to call upon that energy when needed. But something is wrong. You're still tired all the time.

The reason must be that additional demands are being made on your body, but it can't meet them while maintaining a normal activity level. Here are some possible causes for the energy gap.

Multiple sclerosis. This disease, usually referred to as MS, is characterized by an immune reaction in the tissues surrounding brain cells. That reaction consumes excessive amounts of body energy. MS is also characterized by progressive damage to the nervous system, and that leads to progressive muscle weakness, numbness and difficulty with vision.

Fatigue is another primary symptom of the disease.

The illness that most closely resembles MS is CFIDS. The neurological symptoms are strikingly similar, but CFIDS has additional symptoms rare to MS—fever, chills, sore throat and muscle pain. The two illnesses can also be differentiated by laboratory tests.

Perhaps the most difficult task in evaluating fatigue occurs when prominent neurological symptoms exist, which means MS must be considered. It is essential to differentiate MS from CFIDS at the very beginning, since the prognosis of each is unique.

THE CASE OF FATIGUE DUE TO TREATABLE ILLNESS

William was in his thirties when he started to experience unusual periods of fatigue. Over several months they grew more severe and turned into total exhaustion, no matter how much sleep he got.

Not only did William's home life suffer, but his performance at work began to decline. He became depressed and apathetic. Along with the fatigue came periods of weakness and numbness in his arms and legs.

He went to his doctor several times, but there was no improvement. William was still tired all the time.

Then he went blind. His vision loss lasted for just one day, and it finally led to the proper diagnosis. William had MS, multiple sclerosis.

He still has MS, but thanks to medication and treatment, William's fatigue lessened and he is able to function fairly well.

Parkinson's disease and other neurological conditions. Parkinson's disease is a neurological condition that is common among the elderly. Tremors and a shuffling gait are two of its most prominent symptoms. Another is fatigue. Individuals with Parkinson's often have difficulty sleeping—both falling asleep and staying asleep. Their fatigue could be tied to their sleep disorder. But by the time fatigue has become an obvious problem, doctors have already diagnosed Parkinson's by the more noticeable symptoms.

The elderly are also prone to other neurological conditions that cause fatigue, including sleep disorders, anxiety attacks and Alzheimer's disease.

A LOOK AT THE BIG PICTURE

By its very nature, sickness is tiring. Fighting disease requires energy. You have a limited amount of energy, and if you use it to fight illness, there won't be much left to get around on.

Usually taking care of the illness also takes care of the fatigue. But we have seen that there can be complications. Maybe the medicine adds to the fatigue problem. It could be that your illness interferes with your sleep. Perhaps you're depressed about your illness, about your fatigue or about life in general.

People who see their doctor because of severe and persistent fatigue should have a complete examination, including routine blood tests. If there is no obvious medical illness found to explain the fatigue—normal thyroid function, no anemia, no specific infections—then one of the other causes of fatigue becomes much more likely.

CHAPTER 8

Solving the Complex Puzzle of CFIDS

When chronic fatigue immune dysfunction syndrome (CFIDS) strikes, it usually strikes hard, developing suddenly and dramatically disrupting a person's life, often for years. But in some cases (about one person out of four) the start of CFIDS is mild and gradual, building up so slowly that it takes several months—or even years—for the whole symptom pattern to appear.

People with the slow-building type of CFIDS grow accustomed to their fatigue as part of the way they always feel, a natural part of life. For them, pinpointing the exact start of the fatigue is like pinpointing the exact date your gray hair became noticeable or the first time you heard a favorite song.

There are no such questions when CFIDS comes on fast. Its onset is as sudden as a lightning bolt and is especially dramatic in athletes. I know of several professional athletes who became ill in the midst of strenuous training. There had been no warning, no emotional changes that could have explained their symptoms. Certainly they were not lazy, unmotivated or in poor physical condition. They were simply hit with a dramatic illness—CFIDS—that disrupted and rearranged their lives.

This type of lightning strike is often dismissed as "the flu," and indeed, it does feel and act that way. Sometimes victims think they have mononucleosis. But unlike the symptoms of mono, these don't disappear in a few weeks. They persist. Fatigue, headache, sore joints, stomach cramps . . . the whole pattern is easily dismissed as a viral infection. But it won't go away!

This flulike or monolike onset of fatigue is a big clue to CFIDS. Although the actual viruses behind the two diseases may be different, the same mechanisms that cause flu symptoms cause CFIDS symptoms.

Of the many varied factors that can set off CFIDS, the most common is an acute viral infection. But I also know of cases triggered by a vaccine injection, exposure to chemicals or severe stress. Whatever causes CFIDS may lie dormant until some event calls forth the immune response. Then the symptoms show themselves.

Genetics also plays a role. Scientific papers on CFIDS show that several members of the same family may develop the illness simultaneously. Also, over half of those with CFIDS have a history of childhood allergies. Multiple allergies can be thought of as a genetic marker indicating a familial tendency for the immune system to overreact.

JUST TIRED—OR REALLY SICK WITH CFIDS?

The name "chronic fatigue syndrome" is very misleading. It implies that the victim of the illness is tired—but only tired. Nothing is further from the truth. While fatigue may be the most dramatic—and most consistent—symptom, a distinct pattern of other symptoms is what actually identifies CFIDS as a separate disease.

Before we get to those symptoms, it's important to understand that not everyone who has CFIDS has every possible symptom of the illness. True, most CFIDS cases are similar, but different people have different symptoms. New symptoms can develop and old ones disappear, temporarily or permanently.

Generally a disease is first diagnosed by the pattern of symptoms that are present. Then specific laboratory tests confirm the diagnosis. However, there is no specific lab test to confirm CFIDS—yet. The lack of such a test is the basis of the current controversy about the illness.

CLUES TO THE CAUSE

What causes CFIDS? Theories range from nutritional deficiencies to emotions to specific viruses—none of which can be proven. The number of guesses about the cause of CFIDS probably matches the number of researchers investigating the disease.

In the beginning the debate centered on CFIDS itself. Did CFIDS really exist as a separate disease? Eventually the medical community began to accept the fact that it did. Then the debate shifted to the causes. The experts figured it was either a form of depression or a manifestation of the Epstein-Barr virus (EBV), which causes mononucleosis.

Depression. Study after study has shown that CFIDS patients are depressed. Studies also show that they are under stress and sometimes have panic attacks. Since fatigue is a prominent symptom of depression, some researchers took the position that CFIDS was a form of depression. But the basic question remained unanswered: Did CFIDS cause depression, or did depression cause CFIDS?

In fact, the symptom pattern of CFIDS is quite unlike that of clinical depression. To begin with, people with depression do not generally suffer from night sweats, lymph node pain, sore throat and joint pain (typical CFIDS symptoms). Also, the type of fatigue they experience is different. The fatigue of CFIDS is bone crushing and flulike, far from the listlessness and apathy of depression.

Critics of the CFIDS/depression theory noted that almost any illness that leaves individuals debilitated will also leave them depressed. They pointed out that you could use the same questionnaire that was used in the CFIDS/depression survey to show that multiple sclerosis and AIDS are due to depression. Further studies, published between 1985 and 1990, showed that immune system abnormalities present in CFIDS were unlike anything seen in simple depression. Today few informed researchers or physicians can claim that CFIDS is entirely an emotional illness.

Epstein-Barr. Equally flawed was the argument that CFIDS was due to the Epstein-Barr virus. True, early studies of CFIDS sufferers showed that they carried EBV antibodies. But EBV antibodies are *also* found in 95 percent of all healthy adults.

EBV is the cause of most cases of infectious mononucleosis. In its usual form, mono lasts two to three weeks, then resolves itself.

A HEAD-TO-TOE LIST OF CFIDS SYMPTOMS

Here is a list of the many symptoms and the approximate percentage of CFIDS sufferers who experience them.

These are the symptoms that cause the most discomfort, in order of frequency:

- Fatigue or exhaustion (100%)
- Headache (90%)
- Lack of restful sleep (90%)
- Malaise—feeling of the "flu" (80%)
- Short-term memory loss (80%)
- Muscle pain (75%)
- Difficulty concentrating (70%)
- Depression (65%)
- Joint pain (65%)
- Abdominal pain (60%)
- Lymph node pain (50%)
- Sore throat (50%)

Other, less predominant symptoms include:

- Allergies (60%)
- Balance disturbance (30%)
- Bitter or metallic taste (25%)
- Bloating (60%)
- Blurred vision (80%)
- Bouts of diarrhea or constipation (50%)
- Bruising easily (25%)
- Burning during urination (20%)

But anyone who has ever had mono will carry the EBV antibodies for the rest of his or her life. Most adults have had mono, though many cases were so slight that they seemed like a touch of the flu.

In 1985 some researchers also noted that the number of EBV antibodies was greater in persons with CFIDS than in healthy people. But others pointed out that increased antibodies to this virus are associated with a lot of illnesses, such as rheumatoid arthritis, lupus and multiple sclerosis.

Finally, still other studies showed that many people who have CFIDS—especially children—do not have high levels of the virus.

- Chemical sensitivities (25%)
- Chills (30%)
- Clumsiness (30%)
- Dizziness (30%)
- Double vision (10%)
- Earache (20%)
- Eye pain (30%)
- Fainting spells (40%)
- Fever or sensation of fever (65%)
- "Floaters"—seeing spots (30%)
- Flushing rash of the face and cheeks (40%)
- Hair loss (20%)
- Hearing changes (20%)
- Incontinence (10%)
- Insomnia (65%)
- Lightheadedness (75%)
- Loss of sexual drive or performance (20%)
- Muscle weakness (30%)
- Night sweats (50%)
- Numbness and/or tingling in extremities (60%)
- Palpitations (55%)
- Panic attacks (30%)
- Pressure at base of skull (30%)
- Scratchiness in eyes (60%)
- Sensitivity to bright light (80%)
- Shortness of breath (30%)
- Swelling of the extremities or eyelids (20%)
- Weight gain (40%)
- Weight loss (10%)

Now it appears that elevated levels of EBV antibodies are due to the immune system abnormalities involved in CFIDS, not because the virus causes the illness.

During those early years of CFIDS research, elevated levels of various other antibodies were noted in patients with CFIDS. In Great Britain, for example, attention turned to the Coxsackie virus. Scientists there noted that patients with CFIDS had elevated levels of this virus, similar to the elevated levels of the Epstein-Barr virus in America. And it is likely that elevated levels of antibodies to many other different viruses appear in the bloodstreams of people with CFIDS. Why? Because their immune systems aren't working properly.

In the search for a cause of CFIDS—and a cure—still other theories were developed and debated.

Genetics. Some researchers maintain that CFIDS could be caused by a variety of viruses and that those afflicted with it have some sort of genetic defect that blocks their ability to handle these viruses. The fact that family members appear more likely to develop CFIDS favors this theory.

A damaged immune system. Researchers who argued against the genetic defect theory believed that a damaged immune system opened the door to CFIDS. These defects were blamed on everything from chemicals in the environment to mercury in tooth fillings to overuse of antibiotics. But no one has yet identified a specific toxin that consistently causes the disease or its symptom patterns.

Poor nutrition. This is one long-suspected cause of CFIDS. But again, no specific nutritional deficiencies have been proven the culprit. And although taking vitamins may improve some symptoms, supplements are not a cure. CFIDS is not due to a vitamin deficiency. Nutrition is certainly important in treating CFIDS, but it is an unlikely suspect as the source of the ailment.

A new and unknown virus. I personally favor the idea that CFIDS is caused by a specific and still-unidentified virus that defies the immune system. Research now points in that direction, to a virus of the retrovirus family. A promising candidate has shown up in patients with CFIDS. Only time will tell if this virus is the actual culprit.

WHY CFIDS WEARS YOU OUT

Even though we don't know what causes CFIDS, we do know why it makes victims so tired. It's all due to the intricate workings of the immune system itself.

When this system is activated, it produces body chemicals called cytokines, messenger chemicals of a sort. Interleukin-2, for example, is a cytokine made by certain cells of the immune system to alert other cells to the threat of an infection. It prompts cells to grow and divide, thus building an army to ward off the attackers—a marvelous feature of our normal defense network.

But this natural biological action can cause fatigue all by itself. Studies conducted by the National Cancer Institute show that cancer patients treated with interleukin-2 developed severe fatigue and flulike malaise—in fact, they exhibited nearly all the symptoms that have been observed in CFIDS.

Interferons are also cytokines, but of a different sort. These natural antiviral messengers found in certain cells are sometimes used to treat specific viral diseases. But like other drugs, when used to treat certain illnesses, interferons cause fatigue and malaise.

In fact, many of the cytokines being tested as treatments against various other ailments prominently display fatigue as a side effect. CFIDS research that has concentrated on these cytokines has shown that they appear in greater-than-normal numbers in CFIDS patients, compared with levels found in adults without CFIDS.

But why the body's immune system kicks in to produce so many extra fatigue-causing cytokines remains a mystery.

DIAGNOSING KILLER FATIGUE

In 1988 the Centers for Disease Control (CDC) in Atlanta proposed the following criteria for the diagnosis of CFIDS:

1. It must be a new onset of fatigue, severe and disabling enough to cause at least 50 percent reduction in daily activities. This daily fatigue must persist for at least six months.
2. A pattern of numerous other symptoms such as headache, abdominal pain and muscle or joint pain must appear. *Anyone with fatigue but no other symptoms does not have CFIDS.*
3. No other medical illness that prominently features fatigue as a symptom can be present. However, it is not unusual for emotional disturbances or allergies to appear after the onset of CFIDS.

Those criteria were offered to help researchers design studies. But where do they leave the average family practitioner faced with a patient who suspects he or she has CFIDS?

One fundamental question is whether there is such a thing as a *mild* case of CFIDS. Researchers themselves disagree on this point. It is possible that a mild form of the disease, in which the victim's daily activities are not reduced by a full 50 percent, may exist. By the CDC criteria, CFIDS research would not be conducted on such a person. But in my opinion, this is an illness with a spectrum encompassing all grades of fatigue, from the very mild to the very severe.

As for tests to diagnose CFIDS or rule out other conditions, the scenario usually goes something like this:

When a patient suffers from severe fatigue as well as the other accepted CFIDS symptoms but still looks relatively well, the doctor does a physical examination with routine blood tests. And the results may show nothing wrong.

Then the nonroutine tests start, as the doctor delves deeper and deeper into his or her medical textbooks and spends more time looking through medical journals—all of which lead to even more blood tests that come back negative. Meanwhile, doctor and patient alike grow frustrated.

I recommend a simpler and more personal way to make the CFIDS diagnosis:

> If a doctor does not know why a patient is overly tired, and if the patient has a medical record that weighs more than 20 pounds because of all the tests and consultations, providing proof that there is nothing wrong with that patient—then the patient has CFIDS.

This "test" will probably never be accepted by the medical profession, but it works for me.

THE CFIDS PROFILE

In 1985 doctors in Lake Tahoe, Nevada, reported an outbreak of an illness we know as CFIDS. At the time the unusual illness characterized by persistent flulike symptoms bewildered everyone. Because so many of the patients were in their midthirties and affluent, the media labeled the disease "yuppie flu," and the name stuck.

Unfortunately, that name trivializes the devastating effects of CFIDS. Even worse, it creates the impression that only people in their thirties can get it. Here are some typical characteristics of CFIDS patients.

Most people who get CFIDS are in their thirties. But it can strike anyone of any age.

Women are more likely than men to get CFIDS. But when it strikes children, boys and girls are equally at risk.

CFIDS runs in families. My own clinical observation reveals that more than 50 percent of those diagnosed with CFIDS have a family member with a similar pattern of symptoms. That doesn't necessarily mean the other family member will develop a full-blown case of CFIDS, but he or she may have what could be called a minor case.

Hormones appear to play a part. The first symptoms of CFIDS often appear at puberty. It is also possible that the effect of female hormones on the immune system may account for the prominence of women among CFIDS patients. But then again, many immunologic illnesses, from arthritis to multiple sclerosis, are more common in women.

As for CFIDS's reputation as a yuppie syndrome, in my experience, financial status has nothing to do with its onset. But when affluent people with good health insurance develop CFIDS, they go to the doctor and are not satisfied until they get an explanation for their symptoms. That often requires lots of tests and plenty of persistence—plus the refusal to accept "overwork" or "it's all in your head" as a diagnosis. Other people simply don't have the economic or emotional resources to continue searching for the cause of the symptoms.

TREATMENTS ARE EVER EVOLVING

Unfortunately, there is no treatment or medication that stands alone as a cure for CFIDS. It remains a puzzling, painful and sometimes devastating chronic illness. But that doesn't mean that nothing can be done. As with other chronic illnesses like rheumatoid arthritis and lupus, certain treatments can help, even if they don't actually cure. Lifestyle adjustments, proper nutrition, stress reduction and medication may reduce some of the more severe symptoms, sometimes with an encouraging increase in overall activity levels.

One new and exciting treatment now being investigated is a drug called Ampligen. This experimental drug is an antiviral agent not yet approved for general use. But early trials with CFIDS patients show promising results. In the near future, medications that fundamentally alter the course of the illness may be available.

What little is known about CFIDS treatment is based largely upon the experiences of a small number of researchers, and there are few proven methods for doctors to prescribe. The situation seems to be changing, however. New trials are being conducted, and perhaps new and promising treatments will become available within months of this writing.

Because the whole subject of treatment is changing so rapidly, I recommend that people who have CFIDS (or suspect they might) write or call the CFIDS Association, P.O. Box 220398, Charlotte, NC 28222-0398 (800-442-3437). This organization can provide individuals with the latest information. They also publish a quarterly journal.

START WITH THE BASICS

Most physicians agree that certain general measures have a beneficial effect on CFIDS. These are widely employed, and most make good sense.

Pay attention to diet. Doctors encourage people with CFIDS to adopt a highly nutritious diet, supplemented with vitamins, if necessary. One group of researchers found that magnesium injections helped some patients, but the results I've seen have been disappointing. The injections are generally safe but quite uncomfortable.

Reduce stress. While stress does not cause CFIDS, it can certainly aggravate the illness, as it can most other illnesses. Therefore, a program of stress reduction generally cuts back on the severity and intensity of the symptoms. Specific suggestions for stress reduction can be found in chapter 11.

Exercise with caution. Although widely prescribed for defeating fatigue, exercise should be recommended with great caution and monitored carefully in CFIDS cases, since such activity may actually worsen the symptoms in some cases. For more on this, see chapter 16.

Make lifestyle adjustments. A flexible daily schedule is among the most helpful factors in the treatment of CFIDS. For many, taking frequent rest breaks throughout the day enables them to continue with their jobs. A schoolteacher suffering from CFIDS, for example, was able to keep working full-time because she was permitted to nap during her lunch break and one early-afternoon period. She could put in seven or eight hours, provided she had a two-hour rest halfway through the workday. Those who work fixed shifts (on an assembly line, for example) have the most difficult time maintaining their productivity.

HOW NON-CFIDS DRUGS CAN HELP

Until science comes up with a single pill or injection that wipes out whatever causes CFIDS and its symptoms, the best doctors can do is recruit other drugs to deal with specific symptoms and make life easier for the patient.

Help for sleepless nights. Nearly everyone who has CFIDS has trouble sleeping. Merely improving their sleep lessens fatigue, eases muscle and joint pain and helps them concentrate better. All the nondrug treatments mentioned in chapter 9 are worth trying, with or without short-acting benzodiazepines or sleeping pills such as clonazepam (Klonopin). Doctors sometimes prescribe a tricyclic antidepressant, such as doxepin (Sinequan, Adapin), in low doses taken at bedtime.

These medications should be used judiciously and monitored carefully, however. Frequent drug holidays are useful to see if the compounds are still needed and as a strategy for preventing dependency, which is a risk with benzodiazepines.

Relief for pain and depression. Tricyclic antidepressants such as doxepin and amitriptyline (Elavil, Endep, Triavil) are also useful in treating any chronic pain involved with CFIDS, such as headache and joint or muscle pain. People who are in pain are often depressed, and these medications will help elevate their moods, too. Some antidepressants are designed to boost energy. Examples of these are fluoxetine (Prozac), trazodone (Desyrel) and bupropion (Wellbutrin). While these medications may be useful in CFIDS, they should be started at very low doses. In some instances, a CFIDS patient taking antidepressants will feel increased fatigue plus the same unpleasant sensation of agitation that comes from drinking too much coffee. So tell your doctor if you feel *worse* after taking these drugs.

An old antiache standby. My favorite medication for treating CFIDS is aspirin—cheap, plain old aspirin. People are sometimes disappointed by this prescription because aspirin is not very high tech. But certain individuals can get considerable mileage out of this old reliable. Aspirin doesn't cure the feelings of fatigue, but it can relieve the aches and pains, malaise and sometimes headache, making the fatigue more bearable. Abdominal distress or ulcers limit its use in some people, but coated aspirin may resolve that problem for individual patients.

A CFIDS SUCCESS STORY

Nancy was 25, in the prime of her life, with a marvelous husband, family and career that gave her a wonderful sense of fulfillment. She had everything.

Then her life changed. It started with what she thought was a case of the flu—sore throat, achiness, headache and exhaustion. She went to bed, expecting her "flu" to run its course. But it just wouldn't go away. The doctor she consulted after two weeks thought it was a viral infection but took a throat culture to be sure it was not strep throat. It wasn't. Several days later, when Nancy did not feel any better, her physician prescribed antibiotics.

The medication didn't work.

Then fever, chills and muscle pain developed, adding more discomfort to her achy joints. Nancy's eyes burned and became so sensitive that she had to stay indoors during the day and keep the lights dim. Her headaches became intense, and she developed abdominal pains along with the bloating, gas and nausea.

The various symptoms fluctuated from day to day, but the basic pattern stayed the same over the next several months. The only constant was the perpetual fatigue, and it became the center of her life. At one point she had to have a chair moved into the bathroom because she had to sit down to brush her teeth.

As bad as her tiredness was, it got worse after any type of activity. If Nancy went out shopping, for example, she would have to remain in bed for two days to recover.

The months drifted past. She lost her job. The family finances were drained. Her doctor ran dozens of laboratory tests, and all results were normal.

Nonsteroidal anti-inflammatory drugs (NSAIDs) are similar to aspirin and may be useful in treating the headache, joint pain and muscle aches CFIDS patients experience. But they can worsen abdominal pain, and again, caution is advised if a patient has a history of ulcers. You're probably already familiar with some of these drugs, including tolmetin (Tolectin), meclofenamate (Meclomen), flurbiprofen (Ansaid) and ibuprofen (Advil, Motrin, Rufen). For some people, one of these drugs will have little effect but another will be quite helpful, so trying different ones might be

Maybe her problem was depression, her doctor suggested, so he sent her to a psychiatrist. This specialist said Nancy wasn't sick because she was depressed, she was depressed because she was sick!

Several months later Nancy experienced balance problems, memory loss and difficulty in thinking. Since she already suffered from muscle weakness and numbness in her legs, she was tested for multiple sclerosis. That wasn't it, either.

Nancy personally believed she was dying, probably from an undiagnosed cancer. She told her physician about her fears and mentioned the fact that she also had swollen lymph nodes. He told her there could not be a medical cause for all her problems. It was all psychosomatic. Her imagination was running away with her.

She stopped seeing that doctor.

A few months later Nancy heard about chronic fatigue immune dysfunction syndrome (CFIDS) and its many symptoms. Those were *her* symptoms. She went to a physician who was familiar with the disease and had several immune function tests. That was it—she had CFIDS!

The ailment persisted, but at least she knew what she had. It was a real disease. She was actually ill; it wasn't all in her head.

The doctor put her on several different medications that helped ease some of the specific symptoms, even though they did not cure the illness.

About two years later Nancy finally began a slow but steady improvement. Five years after the first symptoms appeared, although she still wasn't completely recovered, Nancy was well enough to go back to work. Her fear and confusion disappeared, and she was able to cope with the remaining symptoms.

of value. Generally narcotics should be avoided, but ketorolac (Toradol) might be given to relieve severe pain.

Help for heavy-duty headaches. Headaches associated with CFIDS can also be treated with several other medications. Migraines, for example, often respond to the class of drugs known as beta blockers, customarily used to quiet heart problems such as racing heartbeats and palpitations. These medications include nadolol (Corgard), atenolol (Tenormin, Tenoretic) and propranolol (Inderal). They should not be used (except with great caution) if there is a history of asthma. But again, this is a matter of trial and error because sometimes these drugs make fatigue worse. In rare situations, acetazolamide (Diamox) has been used effectively to relieve the pressure headaches of CFIDS, but this drug should be prescribed only very cautiously by a physician experienced in its use with CFIDS.

"Smart drugs" for CFIDS? Many people with CFIDS tell me that the inactivity fatigue causes would be tolerable if only they could think! They complain of lack of concentration, short-term memory loss and periods of confusion that can be very frightening. These symptoms are among the most urgent to be addressed. Experimental treatments for cognitive difficulties associated with CFIDS include naltrexone, stimulants (narcolepsy treatments) and other, rarely used neurologic drugs. At this time, unfortunately, very little information is available on their use in treating CFIDS, so they should be used sparingly and with great discretion.

I am convinced that the effective treatment of CFIDS, even a decisive cure, is on the horizon of medical research. As more researchers and practitioners become aware of this devastating disease, the answers will come quickly and minimize the misery of those afflicted.

RECOVERY RATES VARY

The good news is that most people who have CFIDS will regain their energy. It may take as long as five years, but the majority return to a near-normal level of activity. Beyond that, there have been very few reliable medical studies on the long-term outlook. We are hobbled by the requirement of a 50 percent reduction in activity over six months as part of a bona fide diagnosis of CFIDS. As I stated, I am convinced that the illness occurs in milder forms, too. The less virulent the illness is in the first year, the better the chances that the symptoms will be resolved.

A case in point: In the upstate New York epidemic in 1985, 100 people developed CFIDS, meeting the severity criteria of a 50 percent reduction in activity. Another hundred developed the same pattern of symptoms but did not meet the reduced activity measure.

Nearly all of the second group—those with mild cases—recovered completely within five years. In contrast, 70 percent of the first group (those who met the stricter CFIDS criteria) recovered to near-normal function, but many of them continued to have symptoms such as joint pain and headache. Another 15 to 20 percent of that first group persisted with severe symptoms and were disabled. It is unlikely that they will improve much in the future. So it appears that the worse the symptoms are at the start of the disease, the longer the symptoms will last.

A second factor that helps to predict the final result is how abruptly the symptoms occur. People whose symptoms strike out of the blue are more likely to achieve full recovery than those whose symptoms creep up gradually.

Age is a third factor, although there has been little study in this area. Experience suggests that children with CFIDS, particularly those under age ten, are less likely to recover completely than adults. Usually youngsters don't become as ill, and they deal with the symptoms better than adults, but the symptoms don't go away.

Treatment studies are only now beginning. We know that particular treatments improve certain symptoms of CFIDS, but not whether they actually shorten the course of the disease.

THE LONG AND FRUSTRATING WAIT FOR A CURE

For years many physicians denied the existence of such a thing as CFIDS. But then again, back in 1980, many physicians denied the existence of AIDS, too.

CFIDS research is likely to change the face of medicine forever. In the pre-CFIDS medical world, skepticism was always encouraged as a bulwark against quackery, and with good reason. Yet the medical world, protective of its role as arbiter of all medical knowledge, pointedly ignored patients who reported an unusual illness with severe fatigue.

Physicians argued that the illness could not exist in the face of normal results from physical examinations and routine blood tests. They said "mass hysteria" caused thousands of people to describe the same symptoms they read about in newspapers. However, people were reporting these symptoms long before the press ever did.

Today CFIDS is fully recognized as a real illness. A growing number of studies demonstrate the subtle abnormalities in the brain and immune system that are associated with the illness. Over

A WORLDWIDE HEALTH PROBLEM?

CFIDS is probably not a new illness. Over recent years, physicians researching CFIDS have found more than 50 outbreaks of an illness that sounds like CFIDS. In each incident it was called by a different name because the authors of the literature were unaware of similar outbreaks and had not recognized the pattern of symptoms.

Numerous flare-ups of an illness called myalgic encephalomyelitis have occurred around the world since 1930. Perhaps the best descriptions of the illness appeared in the 1950s, when outbreaks were initially linked to polio, at that time a serious public health concern. The initial symptoms were similar: a flulike illness, weakness, headache and sometimes other nervous system changes. But poliomyelitis often progressed to paralysis, while this other strange illness did not, even though the fatigue and numerous symptoms persisted.

"Atypical polio" and "polio-like illness" were the terms used. Many outbreaks were named after the geographic areas of their occurrence, leading to more confusion and inability to make comparisons. But in reading descriptions of these outbreaks, one is struck by the severe persistent fatigue, similar pattern of symptoms and chronic, prolonged course of suffering, all reminiscent of CFIDS. With the decline of

recent years the number of doubting doctors steadily decreased as physicians began to see patients whose lives were devastated by CFIDS.

I remember talking to one family physician who did not hesitate to say that CFIDS was just a fad. As we talked, I described the symptoms, and a light bulb seemed to go on above his head. "That is what Mr. Thompson has!" he exclaimed.

This doctor had struggled for the past year with a patient—an honest, hard-working man—who was very ill. The idea that the unusual illness might be CFIDS had never occurred to the doctor. Once he realized that Mr. Thompson had CFIDS, he suddenly understood what the disease was and recognized it in several other patients. The medical journals rarely described or explained CFIDS, and he had assumed that it was a trivial illness specific to neurotic people.

Now you have seen what a tremendously complicated illness

worries over polio, physicians have forgotten the strange epidemics of an illness that was not polio and was never fully understood.

Part of the great confusion surrounding our present-day understanding of CFIDS is the variety of names accrued to it over the years. In addition to "atypical poliomyelitis" and "myalgic encephalomyelitis," nearly 50 other names have been applied. In a well-studied outbreak on the northern coast of Iceland in 1950, 1,200 persons were affected, and the names "Iceland disease" and "Akureyri disease" were born. An outbreak at the Royal Free Hospital in London was called, sensibly enough, Royal Free disease. However, this habit made it very difficult for physicians to appreciate that this illness was common and occurring worldwide.

In more recent times, awareness of the illness in the United States began in 1985 with the Lake Tahoe outbreak of yuppie flu, later referred to as chronic Epstein-Barr virus disease.

The important thing to remember is that CFIDS is a common illness that has been described in outbreaks all over the world—hardly a vague, psychosomatic illness unique to disgruntled rich people. It is a specific, organic illness that represents a major public health threat. The fact that we do not yet know the cause is no excuse for simply dismissing the disease.

CFIDS is. Proper diagnosis requires that physicians spend more time than usual with their patients. Numerous symptoms need to be explored and many illnesses ruled out by means of extensive testing. But the greatest problem is the frustration experienced by the patient and physician. After six months and $50,000 worth of laboratory tests, one patient still did not know the cause of her numerous disabling symptoms simply because it never occurred to her doctor that she might have CFIDS.

Fortunately, physician awareness is changing, though slowly, and the research seems to be crawling at a snail's pace. There is much we still don't know, and theories about the cause of the illness have yet to be proven. We speculate on the best treatments but have little experimental proof. Yet we do know the pattern of symptoms, and we are coming to see and understand the tremendous impact that CFIDS has on the way we live our modern life.

CHAPTER 9

Sleep Problems? Is That Why You're Bone Tired?

You've been feeling extremely tired all day, every day for months—but why? You're not ill, and you're not working any harder than usual. Your doctor's answer—"Maybe you need more sleep"—seems too simple. Besides, you get enough sleep (eight hours a night), or at least you think so. But you could be wrong on both counts. Your nightly meeting with Morpheus might be dragging you right into exhaustion.

Our language and literature are filled with poems, sayings, bromides, lullabies, rhymes and clichés about the benefits of sleep: "Sleep on it," "Sleep it off," "Sleep like a baby," "He slept the sleep of the just," "You'll feel better after a good night's sleep" and "What you need is sleep."

The way sleep works on us is an unsolved mystery, even among the most dedicated and sophisticated researchers in the field.

Sleep relaxes, rests and renews us, and it flushes our fatigue away. It helps us recover from thousands of life's daily trials and tribulations—but only if it is a *good* night's sleep.

What does that mean? What is a good night's sleep?

Some people wake after eight hours of sleep feeling more tired than when they went to bed; others wake from a half-hour nap feeling completely refreshed. One person might need five hours of sleep a night; another might need ten.

Theories about why we have to sleep range from the metaphysical to the mundane. Some say it is a time of spiritual rejuvenation when the soul contemplates mysteries that cannot even be approached in a conscious state. Others compare it to taking our heads in for servicing, to refill the chemical neurotransmitters of the brain. Many theories fall between these two, and that's probably where the truth is, but we just don't know—yet.

One of the frustrating things about medicine is that the difficult is usually easier to explain and understand than the simple. There are countless medical books, journals and articles explaining exactly how to perform a heart transplant, from the first incision to the last suture. But can someone write out directions that will ensure any person who follows them a good, natural, undrugged and restful night's sleep, night after night after night? No way.

The only thing we know for sure about sleep is that we need it—and that usually we need more than we get.

In terms of chronic fatigue, poor sleep is both a major cause and a major contributing factor. Even if lack of sleep or poor sleep is not the root cause of your energy slump, the odds are that you would still feel better if you could get more of it.

What does sleep actually do for us? Researchers believe it works somehow to conserve our energy and to reestablish our mind/body balance.

We use our muscles, along with our brain, while we're asleep (but less strenuously than when we're awake). So it follows that as we sleep we also use energy, about three-quarters of what we burn during the day. The fact that we use fewer calories gives the body a chance to recharge, to restore the energy balance. Naturally, any sleep disorder puts your body's chance to recharge in jeopardy.

There are numerous other theories about what really goes on when the lights go out.

Some sleep specialists maintain that sleep has little to do with energy recharging. They say the purpose of sleep is to give the mind time to sort through the day's activities. They compare this phenomenon to an office where people are constantly coming in and dropping off paperwork. Unless the door is locked occasionally to stop the flow, there is never time to sort through the papers and file what is important. By allowing our mental office this time to recoup, we wake up with the clear mind and vitality we associate with having had a good night's sleep.

Another theory maintains that while we are awake, our body synthesizes certain chemicals in our nervous system, perhaps as a by-product of conscious experiences. It's the buildup of these chemicals that makes us sleepy. Once we're asleep, the chemicals break down or are distributed through the body. As such, some researchers consider sleep a side effect of wakefulness.

Much of our knowledge about what sleep actually does for us has come from watching people who have been deprived of sleep. Volunteers, usually healthy college students, are paid to stay awake for three or four days and then perform—or try to perform—certain activities. As they perform, they are observed and their body chemistries are monitored and evaluated. The results are compared with how they handle the same tests and tasks after a normal night's sleep.

As with so many expensive and highly structured medical and psychological experiments and testing procedures, the results don't really surprise anyone. They confirm our own experiences after losing sleep because of a crisis at work or with our children. First we feel generalized achiness and a sense of malaise. We are tired, short-tempered and generally miserable. If we're deprived of sleep for too long, our thoughts become disorganized and we lose the ability to concentrate or remember. Performance declines, followed by more and more erratic, even crazy, thinking. We develop paranoid feelings and delusions and perhaps hallucinate. Luckily, most of these symptoms disappear quickly after a good sleep.

PERHAPS YOU NEED LESS SLEEP THAN YOU THINK

Everyone needs eight hours of sleep every night, right? Wrong! No one knows exactly how many hours of sleep anyone needs, but the consensus is that few of us get enough.

All we know for sure is that you need as much sleep as it takes to wake refreshed—whatever that length of time might be. The normal range is from four to ten hours a night, with nearly 10 percent of the population sleeping less than six hours. There is also a great deal of evidence that women generally need to sleep about an hour more than men, especially when pregnant or nursing.

CLUES TO CLOCKING YOUR SLEEP NEEDS

If you use an alarm clock, move it out of sight once it's set. Watching the hours slowly tick away as you battle your insomnia only increases your anxiety.

It's important to know that those who need an alarm clock to wake up are not getting enough sleep. That's the word from researchers at Stanford University's Sleep Disorders Center. Furthermore, they suggest that the length of time it takes you to fall asleep is a valid indicator of whether your sleep time is a factor in the fatigue you experience. (Their findings do not apply to those who have mental, physical or emotional problems that interfere with falling asleep.)

If getting to sleep takes:

- 5 minutes or less, you are probably sleep deprived.
- 15 to 20 minutes, you are probably getting enough sleep.
- Between 5 and 15 minutes, you are a borderline case.

If you're still awake after 20 minutes—get out of bed. You're not ready for sleep.

Researchers agree that seven to eight hours of sleep is most often associated with good health. More than nine hours and less than five are often linked to health problems. (Interestingly, statistics show that people who average eight hours a night are less likely to die of cancer, heart problems or stroke.)

If the start of your fatigue can be linked to the development of a sleeping problem, try to recall how much sleep you got when you felt energetic. That is probably the right amount for you.

But be careful not to sleep too much. For some unexplained reason, getting too much sleep also leaves you tired and groggy. Excessive amounts can even lead to chronic fatigue.

However, no one knows whether health problems are the cause or the consequence of sleep problems. Abnormal sleep patterns could be part of an illness rather than the reason for it.

We know the amount of sleep you need is tied to your age. Senior citizens sleep less than children. But then, senior citizens are more prone to conditions that can interfere with sleep, such as prostate trouble (in men) or bladder problems.

An infant logs an average of 17 hours of sleep a day in scattered naps. And many new parents would say the waking hours seem to be carefully timed to jar you out of a sound sleep.

The older you are, the lighter you sleep. It is perfectly normal for an elderly person to wake up several times during the night. It is also normal to need an alarm clock slightly louder than a dynamite blast to rouse a teenager on a school day.

PUTTING THE "GOOD" IN A GOOD NIGHT'S SLEEP

When it comes to sleeping, quality is much more important than quantity. Half an hour of solid sleep can do as much to renew your energy levels as ten hours of poor, frequently interrupted sleep. Several factors determine sleep quality. The most important one appears to be the REM (rapid eye movement) stage of sleep, which is frequently associated with dreaming. But all the other stages must also occur if the sleeper is to awaken refreshed.

Easy breathing is another essential, since an obstruction (such as blocked sinuses) or the lack of fresh air reduces the amount of oxygen you can take in. This is especially important because you breathe less frequently while you sleep.

Of course, pain, strong emotions or physical illness can also affect sleep patterns. So can lack of exercise. Regular exercise during the day can help combat insomnia. Working out in the evening can leave you too alert or wound up to sleep. You can, however, try some very light exercises at bedtime. Such movements should be the kind that stretch and relax you rather than cause you to work up a sweat.

Only you can determine how much exercise you should do. You don't want to wear yourself out, but you do want to know that you have been moving. And be sure to make it a habit. Regularity and consistency are much more important than intensity.

Sleeping better is only one of the benefits of a regular exercise program. Improved health is another. After a workout, stress and tensions decrease. The type of tiredness you feel may change from nervous exhaustion to muscular fatigue, which makes getting to sleep much easier.

Some who are reluctant to exercise fear that they can't spare the energy. For people who actually have chronic fatigue immune dysfunction syndrome (CFIDS), that could be true. But if you're tired all the time because of insomnia, stress, depression or some other problem, give exercise a try. You could be surprised to find that spending energy will help you feel refreshed and rejuvenated—and able to sleep.

You also need to give some thought to your sleeping quarters. Is your bed comfortable? Firm enough to allow a good night's sleep? Big enough to let you stretch out and get comfortable? Can you roll over and shift positions without running into your bed partner—or falling out of bed?

How about your pillow? Is it too puffy? Too flat? Does it hold your head in a comfortable position? Does it interfere with your breathing? Are you allergic to its stuffing?

Now take a look at your bedroom. Even though we spend more time there than in the kitchen, most people spend more time planning kitchens. Since you will spend approximately one-third of your life in the bedroom, you owe it to yourself—especially to the other two-thirds of your life—to make it as comfortable as possible.

Is it quiet? Does your bed partner snore? Would earplugs help? Or would they make you nervous, afraid that you'd miss an important phone call or a cry for help from one of your children?

Is your bedroom too bright? Would wearing a sleep mask help? Is the room too stuffy? Too breezy? Too hot? Too cold?

If your bedroom is conducive to sleep but you still can't nod off, here are several more measures to try.

Tell yourself that the day is over. What's done is done. Anything else will have to wait until tomorrow. If a major problem keeps bothering you, ask yourself this simple question: "Is there anything I can do right now—at this very moment—that will have any actual effect on it?" If the answer is yes, do it; if not, promise yourself you'll get to it as soon as you are able to do something about it.

Try a glass of warm milk. It contains L-tryptophan, a substance that acts to encourage sleep. While you're at it, consider limiting caffeine to the hours before 6:00 P.M. And don't forget, caffeine is found not only in coffee but also in tea, cola and chocolate, plus a number of medications such as over-the-counter painkillers.

Soak in a hot tub. This is a really easy way to wind down (but don't make the water so hot that you turn pink).

Read something relaxing. Try a good romance novel, for example, or a hobby magazine.

Read something boring. You can, for example, save up all the life insurance offers that come in the mail or annual stock reports you receive and keep them in a stack by the side of your bed for such an occasion.

Get into bed. Turn out the lights, close your eyes and let your mind go blank.

Tense and then slowly relax each muscle group in your body, one by one. Start with your toes and your feet, and work your way up to your eyes. Accompany this with slow and steady breathing. Slowly inhale through your nose, hold it for five seconds, and then slowly exhale through your mouth.

Get a relaxation tape and play it quietly next to your bed. This can be soothing music or a prerecorded tape that talks you through relaxation exercises. If you prefer, a tape of nature sounds—a babbling brook or rolling ocean waves—might do the trick.

Watch late-night TV. The less interesting the program, the better.

Pretend that it's really 7:00 A.M. and you have to get out of bed now, immediately. You have to get up. Up! Up! Up! Right now! You'll probably go right to . . . zzzzzzzz.

TO NAP, OR NOT TO NAP

Thomas Alva Edison, the man who invented the light bulb and made staying up all night convenient, was a world-class nap taker.

Historians say that Edison would lie down and take a nap whenever he felt tired. Then after a half hour or so, he would wake up fully refreshed and ready to go back to work, be it 3:00 P.M. or 3:00 A.M. As a result, he rarely slept more than four or five hours a night. But Edison's singular sleep patterns obviously did not interfere with his creativity or ability to work—the man held more than 1,000 patents!

Architect, engineer and writer R. Buckminster Fuller was another genius who preferred his sleep in small doses. His biographer notes that Fuller would work for about six hours and then, at the first sign of fatigue, he would lie down for a half-hour nap. In that way, he could go for long periods on a total of two hours' sleep a day.

In the biography *Bucky,* by Hugh Kenner, the architect explained his system: "I was trying to find out how much I could get done and noticed that a dog, when he gets tired, simply lies down and sleeps. So it could be that if the minute you're tired you lie down, you'll need far less sleep."

Fuller continued that pattern until he was into his seventies, then he sensed the need for more sleep—five or six hours a night—to keep up his creative energy.

Many people rely on naps to help them keep going. In Spain, Mexico and other hot-climate countries, taking a siesta is a natural part of life and business.

In the 9-to-5 world most of us inhabit, increasing numbers of people manage to snatch a half-hour nap after lunch, and they feel the better for it all afternoon. Experts on sleep and attentiveness have found that a midday nap can refresh even normal, healthy workers, especially those with demanding jobs. Inexplicably, however, some people see napping as a sign of weakness.

The truth about napping is simple. Babies sleep when they are tired because it is natural and makes them feel good. Senior citizens do the same. The fact is that a short nap after lunch or dinner, or both, revives them for the rest of the day, and that's reason enough to take those naps.

Some people complain that napping during the day interferes with a restful sleep that night and throws off their daily routine. If this happens to you, don't nap.

HOW THE NATURAL SLEEP CYCLE GOVERNS YOUR REST

Victims of chronic fatigue cannot afford to ignore the vital sequence of sleep's progress through the night. The key to excessive tiredness might lie in the interrupted timetable of nature's predetermined program for REM and non-REM sleep.

REM sleep. Normal sleep is divided into two main classes: REM (rapid eye movement) sleep and non-REM sleep. Perhaps you have observed someone in REM sleep. Even with their eyelids closed, it's obvious that their eyes are moving back and forth, as if they were watching a tennis match.

According to EEG (electroencephalogram, or brain wave) readings, the brain is really working in REM sleep. In fact, readings during REM sleep are similar to those taken while someone is awake. Even though we are only in the REM stage for 20 percent of

DEAR DIARY . . . DETAIL YOUR PERSONAL SLEEP HABITS

Keep a notebook by the side of your bed and use it to record how well or how poorly you sleep.

Note the time you get into bed. If you can't sleep, make a note every half hour as long as you're awake and record how you spend that half hour: reading, planning tomorrow's activities, reviewing your day, praying, meditating and so forth.

If you wake up during the night, record it. If you know why you woke up, write that down, too.

In the morning estimate what time you fell asleep—10 minutes after your last note, 15, 20? How well did you sleep? How do you feel?

Figure out how many hours you actually slept. Many people are surprised by the answer. Usually they slept longer than they thought.

But the diary is not limited to what happens in bed. Keep a record of your caffeine intake and when you consume it. Do you find it easier to fall asleep on nights when you've had less caffeine? Does the time at which you take caffeine affect how fast you fall asleep? Record anything else that might affect your sleep: alcohol, a fight with your spouse, stress, medications and so forth.

The longer you keep a sleep diary and the more you use it, the clearer you'll be about what helps and what interferes with your sleep.

When you start working on your insomnia this way, you should see a difference within a few days. A sleep log helps you remember how long you tossed and turned and when you actually got to sleep. You'll feel encouraged by any progress that you make because you can see it in writing.

Keep the diary going for as long as you need it.

our sleep time, this is when we do most of our dreaming. In sleep-lab experiments, researchers woke people as soon as they started REM sleep, not allowing them to dream. Then the subjects were allowed to sleep as long as they wanted through the other stages of sleep. However, the loss of their REM sleep state—and of their dreams—caused these people severe emotional difficulties, which remained until they were allowed to catch up on their dreaming.

Non-REM sleep. Non-REM sleep is the other kind of sleep. Your eyes aren't moving, and your brain is relatively inactive. Here is what you do when you are sleeping but not dreaming.

Stage 1. This is a transition stage. It doesn't last very long. You are in a very light sleep.

Stage 2. You are just beginning to drift into a sound sleep. The different EEG waves generated by the brain begin to slow down. Breathing becomes deep and rhythmic. But if you wake up while in this stage, you will do so quickly and be relatively alert.

Stage 3. You are getting deeper and deeper into your sleep. If you were hooked up to an EEG, it would be producing large, smooth waves.

Stage 4. This is the deepest level and probably the most restorative. It's hard to wake you up when you're in this stage, and when you do get up, it takes you a long time to become fully alert.

Going through the stages of non-REM sleep plus REM sleep is called a sleep cycle. A cycle runs for about an hour and a half, with the dream state lasting between five and ten minutes. During a normal night's sleep, you go through several cycles.

While all types of sleep are important, sleep-lab research indicates that people who need less sleep usually fall sound asleep more quickly. Overall, people who get by on five or six hours a night spend as much time in stages 3 and 4 and REM sleep as do persons who sleep eight or nine hours a night. Somehow they manage to do without stages 1 and 2.

It's fairly easy to see when someone is in stage 4 sleep, especially if it's your bed partner or one of your children. They breathe very deeply and slowly. If they snore, this is when it will be the loudest. They don't move around very much.

After stage 4, people go back into REM sleep. That's when they dream and are more likely to move around. Their breathing is shallower and quieter. You might even see their eyes move behind their closed eyelids as they follow the action of their dreams.

Noninsomniacs wake up anywhere from two to six times a night, but usually for only a few brief moments. They rarely remember it in the morning.

When insomniacs do fall asleep, they, too, wake up anywhere from two to six times a night. But they have a tendency to stay awake longer, become more alert and remember it more. Sleep studies show that insomniacs spend less total time in REM sleep than otherwise healthy people.

Many sleep researchers blame sleep-cycle abnormalities for much of the daytime fatigue that people experience. They have identified a number of sleep disorders. Here are the common ones.

INSOMNIA: THE NIGHTMARE OF SLEEPLESS NIGHTS

Insomnia won't kill you, but it sure can make life miserable.

Approximately one-fourth of all Americans consider themselves insomniacs. Nearly half of adults have intermittent periods of insomnia, and all of us have experienced an occasional night of pillow-punching wakefulness—women more than men. The problem increases with age.

"Insomnia" means different things to different people. Experts define it as the inability to fall asleep within 30 minutes of getting into bed. Other symptoms include poor sleep quality, getting less sleep than normal, waking up and staying awake for more than 30 minutes during the night and feeling tired during the day.

You know what it's like. You lie in bed, tossing and turning, your mind racing, hoping for sleep to come to switch your thoughts off. You count sheep, you pace the floor. Your mind magnifies every problem you have and even invents some new ones to worry about. Then it starts to project the problems you'll have tomorrow because you'll be too tired from lack of sleep to get anything done—and you have so much to do! The cycle can last until morning, and if that happens night after night, you have chronic insomnia, which we'll look at a little later.

In case you didn't know, the single greatest cause of insomnia is stress. In fact, some researchers see insomnia as a form of stress. Sleep studies show that the same body mechanisms that are at work in stress disorders are present in insomnia. At the very least, inability to fall asleep at will can leave you angry or frustrated.

Stress is also the most important factor in evaluating insomnia. As we'll see in chapter 10, reducing stress is a better way to cure insomnia than any sleeping pill you can take. Insomnia is also closely linked with emotional problems such as chronic anxiety and depression, which will also be discussed in other chapters.

Many people become insomniacs because they never get on a regular sleep schedule. In fact, some people actually develop the insomnia habit.

Insomnia's symptoms are easy to diagnose. The most obvious one, difficulty getting to sleep, affects three out of four insomniacs. The rest can get to sleep—but they can't stay asleep. They wake up early and stay awake. Even though women tend to have more trouble falling asleep, men are more likely to wake up and stay up in the middle of the night.

It's hard to separate cause and effect with insomnia. It's intertwined with stress, and they feed off each other. It can become a vicious cycle that can lead to chronic insomnia.

Chronic insomnia. If night after night goes by and you continually have trouble falling asleep—or staying asleep—you have chronic insomnia. Although it can occur at any age, chronic insomnia usually hits before 40. Most sufferers can trace it to a single traumatic event or stressful period that caused sleeplessness, and the insomnia became a behavior pattern that lingered even after the triggering problem passed.

Chronic insomniacs have higher heart rates during sleep than healthy people. Their body temperatures are higher, and blood circulation in their arms and legs is reduced. Blood tests show that levels of certain chemicals, known as catecholamines, are higher than they should be. All this means that chronic insomniacs are in a state of perpetual activation.

The autonomic nervous system that prepares us for life-threatening crises (the fight-or-flight mechanism) is on duty throughout the night and is reflected in an insomniac's body chemistry. Of course, this is the direct opposite of the emotional and physical states that encourage a good night's sleep.

An overactive autonomic nervous system uses up a lot of energy. Instead of sleep washing over us and restoring our composure and energy, our sleep is light, tense and easily disturbed. We wake up exhausted and unrested, with little energy to face the new day.

Pseudo-insomnia. Insomniacs would dream of going to sleep—if they could get to sleep long enough to dream. Pseudo-insomniacs are people who do go to sleep—but dream that they're awake!

It's not a common condition, but it does exist. People complain that they are tired all the time because they can't get to sleep.

When they are monitored, observers see that they do fall asleep. But when they wake up, they are sure they have been up all night, tossing and turning. Like most other types of insomnia, pseudo-insomnia is probably stress-related.

A LOOK AT DRUGS AND ALCOHOL AS SLEEP AIDS

"It's 3:00 A.M. I haven't been to sleep yet. Should I take a pill? How about a drink?" Most people have asked themselves such questions more than once. Pills and potions can serve as a good short-term answer—or as a dangerous and unsatisfying long-term solution.

Those over-the-counter remedies that induce sleep are most commonly used. Although they do have some sedative action, technically these preparations are not sleeping pills. That means they are not as dangerous but also not as effective. Such products usually contain one of the antihistamines found in cold or allergy capsules that have drowsiness as a side effect, which makes them good sleep inducers.

When you move into sleeping pills that require a prescription, you're dealing with drugs that are powerful and dangerous. Sleeping pills always carry the threat of addiction—that is, you can't get to sleep without them, or you need higher and higher doses to do the job.

The way sleeping pills kill is very simple: Take too many, and your brain shuts down. You forget to breathe.

Some sleeping pills are more dangerous than others. There are two main types of pills: barbiturate-based sedatives, which make you relax and calm your excitement; and benzodiazepine-based hypnotics, which produce drowsiness and get you in the mood to sleep.

When you use alcohol on a regular basis to help yourself fall asleep, you're facing another potential problem—alcoholism. While alcohol is a stimulant when you take it in small doses, it has a strong sedative—almost narcotic—effect in larger amounts. But an alcoholic stupor is not the same as sleep in terms of rest and revitalization. Those who drink to induce sleep are courting addiction to a substance that actually is a countermeasure to their needs.

Taking pills and potions to sleep is complicated by your body's tendency to build up a tolerance to them. So it takes more and more to put you to sleep—usually for shorter and shorter periods. Then you may choose to take yet another dose to do the trick. By this time you're taking a pill to cure the very problem created by the pill!

At a certain point larger doses don't really put you to sleep. They make you pass out. And if you pass out, you don't really wake up. You come to. When you do, if you're very, very lucky, all you'll have is a hangover.

When you've reached the point where you need pills or potions on a regular basis, the only solution, as crazy as it may sound to your 3:00 A.M. mind, is to do without. If that seems impossible, consult your doctor or one of the numerous self-help groups such as Alcoholics Anonymous or Narcotics Anonymous. Some people are under the mistaken impression that only street people can be alcoholics or drug addicts. The simple fact is, if you cannot sleep without drugs (whether they're prescription or not) or alcohol, you have a problem. The support groups can help you.

In situations like the following, the benefits of sleep aids justify the risks, provided the drugs are taken for a limited time and under a doctor's supervision: to survive a severe emotional trauma; to cope with specific sleep disorders; to reset your body's biological clock; and to cope with CFIDS-connected sleep problems that aggravate the chronic fatigue. Sleeping pills help make life more bearable in such cases. Since people with CFIDS might have to be on the medication for a long time, they should take regular drug holidays. Even though a break will cause short-term sleeping problems, it helps avoid long-term addiction and other related problems. There is more about this in chapter 8.

The key point to remember about sleeping pills is this: In some cases they can be a valuable tool. But over the years they have caused a lot more problems than they have solved.

INSOMNIA CURES: WHAT WORKS FOR *YOU?*

When Winston Churchill had trouble falling asleep, he used to switch beds. Charles Dickens thought it helped to have the head of his bed face due north. And Alexander Dumas followed his doctor's orders to stand under the Arc de Triomphe and eat an apple every morning at 7:00 A.M. They were all insomniacs.

Only Dumas had the right idea—or at least his doctor did. Curing the famous French writer's insomnia had nothing to do with standing under the Arc de Triomphe or eating an apple. It had to do with getting out of bed first thing in the morning and then staying up all day. One cause of Dumas's insomnia had been his lack of a regular schedule. We all need some structure in our lives.

One of the best cures for insomnia is to get out of bed at the same time every morning and stay up for 16 hours. Then go to bed. Whether or not you sleep, make sure you are up and out of bed at the regular time. The first week is the hardest, but unless your insomnia is stress-related or has a medical cause, the odds are that you will get back into a normal sleep routine.

Other people are forced out of their normal sleep habit by their jobs or lifestyles. For example, some suffer from sleep displacement. These proverbial night people seem to come alive only after the sun has set; even if they do go to bed early, they can't fall asleep until dawn. They have two choices: to move into a time zone that corresponds to their body clock, or to reset their body clock. To reset, they go to bed a little later every day, then get out of bed after eight hours—no matter what. Eventually this puts them back on schedule.

People who develop sleep displacement because of their work hours have a real problem: Shift work eventually erodes their capacity both to sleep and to stay awake. (See chapter 17 for more on shift worker's fatigue.)

QUIETING RESTLESS LEGS SYNDROME

A mild form of restless legs syndrome affects more than 5 percent of the population, but for those with more serious cases, it is a major cause of insomnia. It can lead to daytime sleepiness and, if it goes on long enough, chronic fatigue.

The main symptom is an uncomfortable "crawling" sensation in the legs, which begins soon after lying down to rest. The legs may begin to twitch and jump with uncomfortable or painful muscle contractions, sometimes quite dramatically. You may have to sit up and rub or stretch your muscles, sometimes even walk around the room to quiet them. Most sufferers have a rough time actually getting to sleep. Those who do sleep wake up frequently due to muscle contractions. Sufferers might not remember that they woke up, but their bed partners will.

Many researchers consider the syndrome to be an exaggeration of the sleep starts that nearly all of us (or our bedmates) have at times while just drifting off to sleep. These sudden muscle contractions are normally not uncomfortable, and as a rule they do not awaken us. The syndrome is common in many neurological and muscle diseases and tends to worsen with caffeine consumption, smoking, temperature changes and, for reasons no one really understands, pregnancy. It has also been observed as a side effect of certain medications.

Restless legs syndrome is easy to spot in a sleep laboratory because monitoring wires are routinely connected to the legs. But if you talk to your doctor about your insomnia, the odds are the subject won't come up, unless your bed partner is part of the discussion. He or she is the one who is kept awake or wakened by your thrashing legs. (You might not even be conscious of your own sleep disturbance, though you might feel tired next day.) Aside from finding another place to sleep, your partner can try to help you lick the problem by encouraging you to do some light leg exercises before bedtime, use hot bandage soaks for your legs or take an over-the-counter benadryl preparation for relief.

SNORING: NOT JUST A NUISANCE

"Apnea" is a medical term that means interrupted breathing; sleep apnea occurs when you stop breathing while you're asleep. It is a fairly common but rarely recognized problem. In fact, sleep apnea is among the most prominent yet underdiagnosed causes of chronic fatigue.

The brain controls both your sleep pattern and your breathing. Any disturbance that causes intermittent gaps in the breathing pattern (brain injuries, infections, tumors, strokes) is called central apnea and is relatively rare. Obstructive sleep apnea (breathing problems caused by any obstructions in the upper airways) is much more common.

The muscles in the back of the throat are really respiratory muscles, and poor tone or too much relaxation of these muscles causes the airways to narrow. This interferes with the free flow of air during sleep—the setting for sleep apnea. A number of different factors will aggravate the condition: obesity; colds, flu or other upper respiratory infections; throat tissues that are swollen because of smoking or allergies; or a deviated nasal septum. Any of these,

THE CASE OF THE MAN WHO COULDN'T STAY AWAKE

Marty was 47 years old, happily married with three children and had a good job. He didn't have any major worries. He was just tired all the time and had been for years.

He knew it wasn't due to overwork because he felt exhausted even while on vacation. Marty knew it must be tied to his sleeping pattern because he even woke up tired. Coffee helped him get through the morning, but he spent the rest of the day fighting sleep.

His doctor noted that Marty was anxious, mildly overweight and a smoker—characteristics typical of people with sleep problems. Marty also told the doctor he woke up with severe headaches that lasted an hour or two. A routine physical drew a blank, but the doctor prescribed sleeping pills.

Two weeks later Marty was back, more exhausted than ever. He had even missed several days of work. The morning headaches were worse and accompanied by hangovers, caused by the sleeping pills.

Marty was referred to a sleep specialist, who asked detailed questions. One was about snoring, a subject the family doctor hadn't raised and one neither Marty nor his wife had mentioned.

Marty was a terrible snorer—always had been. In fact, he and his wife had had separate bedrooms for the past five years because of it. His 12-year-old son called it Olympic-quality snoring. Once the neighbors complained about the snores that floated through the open windows and across the backyard.

The specialist also learned that Marty didn't breathe regularly when he slept. The snores would be interrupted by gasps and long pauses, followed by his turning over and

alone or in combination, may constrict the upper airways so that the lungs do not get enough air while the rest of the body sleeps.

Overweight middle-aged men who also have high blood pressure are typical sufferers of sleep apnea. One of the most noticeable symptoms in the vast majority of cases is snoring—incredibly loud snoring. The snores may be interrupted by gasps, pauses and sometimes jerking motions as the body struggles for air. Sometimes beginning to snore again. Occasionally Marty would jump up in his sleep after a long pause in his breathing.

A sleep study confirmed the specialist's suspicion that Marty suffered from sleep apnea.

The muscles of Marty's airways were weak, so when he slept on his back, as he usually did, the soft palate hung down and the inhaled air made it vibrate, causing the loud snoring. His obesity and smoking made it worse, as did the sleeping pills. But the real problem was that Marty couldn't get enough air as he slept because his airways would narrow. Sometimes he would stop breathing for 10 or 15 seconds. This woke him up—more than 300 times a night—as he tried to breathe.

Sleep apnea also explained Marty's morning headaches. They were due to the impaired exchange of oxygen for carbon dioxide. The excess carbon dioxide that accumulated caused the pain. After an hour or two of normal breathing in the morning, the carbon dioxide levels returned to normal and the headaches disappeared.

There were several elements involved in Marty's treatment: He stopped smoking, gave up alcohol and sleeping pills and began a weight-loss program. He trained himself to sleep on his side, propped with cushions to prevent him from rolling onto his back. He was also treated with an oxygen flow device that kept his blood oxygen levels in the normal range while he slept.

Slowly Marty began to improve. In a second "sleep checkup" six months later, Marty woke up only 25 times. The real evidence of improvement lay in his renewed sense of vitality and energy; he no longer felt sleepy during the day. His performance skyrocketed, a development his co-workers attributed to weight loss. But the actual reason for the change was that, for the first time in years, Marty was able to sleep and breathe at the same time.

the sufferer will sit upright in bed in order to begin breathing again. As soon as normal breathing resumes, the patient goes back to sleep—until the next time.

An infant with sleep apnea can't sit up to begin breathing again. That's why some researchers believe that this condition is a major cause of sudden infant death syndrome (SIDS), also known as crib death.

Adults with apnea rarely remember having to wake up to breathe. Their bed partners often notice it but don't realize what is going on. They are usually just relieved that the victim has stopped snoring for even a little while.

Even though they think they have slept through the night, sleep apnea victims do not get either a long enough or a deep enough sleep. It is light and constantly interrupted by the need to breathe. As a result, they wake up far from rested. Daytime fatigue and sleepiness, compounded by crankiness, are common consequences and may be severe enough to cause problems at both work and home. Sufferers can also fall asleep at odd moments during the day, such as while driving or operating dangerous machinery. Sufferers who have poor circulation as well are in even greater danger. Other symptoms include morning headaches, sweating during sleep and frequent night trips to the bathroom (due to the frequent wakening rather than any urinary tract problems).

Sometimes the condition is a complication of a disease such as muscular dystrophy or hypothyroidism. Nocturnal asthma attacks, which occur primarily during sleep, are also frequently related to sleep apnea. Alcohol, sleeping pills or medications that relax muscles along the respiratory tract may either cause or aggravate this condition.

Obstructive sleep apnea must be diagnosed in sleep laboratories and treated. If you have the symptoms, discuss them with your own doctor first. In some cases sleep apnea can be cured by a lifestyle change: losing weight, stopping smoking, quitting drinking or changing medication. One woman noticed a marked decline in her husband's snoring—and an increase in restfulness—when her mate cut out alcohol and lost ten pounds.

NARCOLEPSY: THE URGENT NEED TO SLEEP—*NOW!*

Narcolepsy is a sleep disorder that causes pronounced fatigue, and its specific symptoms are frequently missed by physicians. A rare condition that strikes only 1 person in 5,000, it is readily treated. The symptoms are so specific that those with narcolepsy will know if they have it.

The primary symptom, irresistible sleepiness, occurs during the day. You fall asleep at awkward, inopportune or potentially dangerous moments—such as in the middle of a conversation or while driving a car! The victim is forced by nature to sleep for ten minutes to an hour. In general, the sleepiness and fatigue persist throughout the day. You can't think straight or perform your job very well.

In one prominent symptom of narcolepsy, called sleep paralysis, the victim awakes but cannot move or talk. This is terrifying. Many victims are convinced that they have died.

Victims of narcolepsy-based chronic fatigue may be afraid to mention these "crazy" symptoms to a doctor.

Narcolepsy is a genetic illness—that is, it tends to run in families. Most victims are men, and the condition is often triggered by some severe stress or psychological trauma. A specific blood test for a genetic component in narcoleptics has been developed to aid in the diagnosis.

Narcolepsy must be treated and monitored by a specialist in sleep disorders. A number of drugs can halt the attacks of sleep and paralysis and remove the daytime tiredness so that the victim can lead a relatively normal life.

THE SLEEP LAB

Most medical labs are places where body tissue or fluid samples are sent for study. A sleep lab requires the whole body.

People are sent to sleep labs—scientific laboratories with beds—for a one- or two-night stay if their doctors suspect a sleep disorder.

Patients sleep through the night in comfortable beds while wearing wires attached to the scalp. These wires connect them to an EEG to record the brain's electrical activity. Other instruments will record respiratory rate, muscle movement and oxygen intake.

The process is a lot easier than it sounds. After all, the only thing you have to do is sleep—the lab staff does the real work, feeding continuous EEG readings into a computer for analysis.

The EEG's brain wave activity measurement is the key. Researchers have noted several distinct phases of brain wave activity in normal sleep. The EEG records the different sleep stages, all of which are necessary for proper rest, and can help pinpoint what stage you might be having problems with.

CHAPTER 10

Stress, the Painful Partner of Fatigue

All too often stress and fatigue go hand in hand. Think of total exhaustion and job burnout, just two results of too much stress.

Along with its role as the most common single cause of excessive fatigue, stress causes or aggravates a wide spectrum of medical conditions, which can in turn bring on or worsen fatigue. These include heart disease, high blood pressure, insomnia, back pain, stomach problems, hemorrhoids, ulcers and menstrual problems. Prolonged stress also weakens the body's immune system, leaving us open to more frequent and more serious colds, infections, flu and other illnesses that also take their toll in energy.

In other words, even if stress isn't what's making you tired, it's certainly not *helping* matters.

SOLVING THE PUZZLE OF STRESS

Here is an ailment that is neither a germ nor a virus, neither an injury nor an infection. And even though it is not contagious, if everyone around you has it, there's a very good chance that you'll develop it, too.

Simply put, stress is the reaction of your body and mind to the various social, physical and emotional pressures of modern life.

It is impossible to avoid stress and still live, love, work and play in today's world. Sickness, busy schedules, crime, politics, traffic, pollution, fragmented rest periods, the pressure to achieve, the need to be successful, troubled finances—they all conspire to cause stress.

Stress leads to worry, and worrying is hard work. It takes a lot of energy.

Some people argue that stress is a modern affliction. But, in fact, Cro-Magnon humans were stressed, too, and for many of the same reasons we are: the pressure to maintain an unbroken food supply; the need to find and preserve warm shelter; the danger of physical or psychological injury from others. Stress is a basic feature of the human condition. The way we handle stress is what governs its longtime effect on us.

Stress is a reaction to a threat, an emergency or pressure. We feel it when we apply for a job, when we anticipate going on a vacation or trip, when we get yelled at or snubbed, when we skid while driving or when we see a two-year-old child lean out a window.

In cases like these, stress is both normal and necessary. It produces the fight-or-flight response, which gives us the strength and energy to react, respond, fight or run away.

A certain degree of stress is good for us. It keeps us sharp and gives us an edge, an added alertness we sometimes need. But when our system is overloaded with stress, we tend to surrender to it by becoming dull and apathetic and giving in to exhaustion.

The first symptom of a normal stress response is an energy surge—a sudden burst of strength, a rush of adrenaline. Stress allows people to perform almost superhuman feats of strength in times of danger: A mother lifts a car off of her child after a wreck; a father tears a door off the hinges to rescue his family from a fire; a small child pulls a much larger adult to safety.

THE CHEMISTRY OF STRESS

Energy seems to come from out of nowhere in times of stress. In fact, it comes out of the energy reserves stored in body tissues and produced by body chemistry.

THE CASE OF PERFECTIONISM-INDUCED STRESS

Martha held a full-time job as a medical secretary, worked a lot of overtime, managed a family with three teenagers and kept house. She did everything as well as possible. Also, she was always very tired.

Her time was never her own. When she wasn't working, she acted as her children's chauffeur. She also had to make sure that her husband got his dinner on time. She did a lot, and everything had to be just right.

Suddenly Martha began to have outbursts of anger for no reason. Then she and her husband started to grow apart. She complained of being under constant stress, and she resented his demands.

But when she actually had time for herself, all for herself, she would find something that she just had to do—for other people.

She was exhausted and had frequent headaches and a perpetually upset stomach. She relied on coffee to get her going and sedatives to calm her down.

Somehow she was able to cope with her hectic schedule. What she couldn't handle was her conviction that she was a failure. No one appreciated her efforts. No matter how hard she tried, nothing seemed to work out. When she was inactive, the feeling of failure was worse than ever, so she tried to cope by working even harder.

The classic fight-or-flight response, the instinct for self-defense or escape called into play by stress, is actually located in the brain and in the adrenal glands just above the kidneys. When the brain perceives a threat, it alerts the adrenal glands to release the hormone adrenaline and other chemicals that speed up our heart rate, force us to take deeper breaths, put us into a heightened state of alertness and give us the burst of energy vital for necessary action.

These physiological changes increase the amount of oxygen in the blood and carry it to the tissues where it is needed to meet the emergency. This changes the way blood circulates. More blood goes to the heart, brain and muscles, and less blood circulates through the skin. That's why we have cold, clammy and sweaty palms during an emergency.

Martha's goal was to be perfect, but somehow she never quite made it. She saw anything that went wrong as her fault. It didn't matter whether anyone blamed her. She blamed herself for being less than perfect.

She'd been that way all her life. Her earliest childhood memories were of being scolded. When her parents ended their stormy marriage, Martha was only six. She felt that the divorce was her fault, too. If she had been a better child, she kept telling herself, her parents would have stayed together. The way she saw it, their divorce was just the first disappointment in a life filled with failures.

Martha finally realized that she needed help, and she began to explore her feelings of inadequacy and guilt with a psychotherapist. Over the next few months, the links between her childhood frustrations and her current feelings began to emerge.

With her newfound knowledge, Martha was able to explore stress-reduction techniques, cut her coffee consumption and stop using tranquilizers. More important, she began to improve her self-image, seeing herself as an intelligent, capable and loving person, not a martyr and a slave. She also quit blaming herself for everything that went wrong.

Martha changed her self-image and her lifestyle and stopped pushing herself so hard. She no longer accepted responsibility for anyone else's actions and actually took time out for herself. Eventually her fatigue became a thing of the past.

The increased blood flow to the brain makes us more alert. In an emergency, we can go from sound sleep to complete alertness in seconds; we think fast, though our thinking is jumbled. In times of severe stress, the mind can't deal with complex issues. It searches for the simplest and fastest response to a pressing situation.

Sometimes that reaction is counterproductive, but it's hard to convince someone having an adrenaline rush to stop what he or she is doing or to do it differently. That's why the greatest danger in saving a drowning person is to let that person get a hold on you. A drowning victim is more likely to kick and grab and fight than to cooperate in being pulled to safety.

All this extra blood circulation, tension and adrenaline also hits the intestines, so during periods of high stress we feel that our stomach is tied in knots. Like animals that sometimes relieve themselves when trapped and frightened, we might have a sudden urge to urinate, or we might develop diarrhea or start vomiting. This, too, is natural. The body is preparing itself to run away by getting rid of excess weight.

When the emergency is over, we are exhausted, drained. This is the normal recovery phase of a stress response. We've used up enormous reserves of energy, and now we must pay for it.

If you stay in that stressed state after the threat has passed, it can lead to many things, but sleep is not one of them. That's why stress is such a common partner to insomnia.

The body has only so much energy to spend when the fight-or-flight response kicks in. And the body can't judge whether it's facing a real emergency or just another worry grown large, but when that response takes over, nothing is held back.

The fight-or-flight response that can save your life in a real emergency can also drain your life if it persists too long. Drugs like cocaine or amphetamines induce that state of heightened awareness and strength. If you use them, you're committing suicide on the installment plan, paying in larger and larger amounts of energy stores the more you use drugs. The last payment could be a killer. But hostility, anger, worry and other negative emotions can be just as deadly.

RELIEF FOR CHRONIC STRESS

The body simply can't put up with perpetual stress, so it makes accommodations, often by ignoring the stress. That's why people with physically dangerous jobs seldom develop chronic stress. They usually adjust to both the job and the pressure. Otherwise they leave the job voluntarily or are fired for poor performance, unless an accident forces them to quit.

It's not the dangers that do the damage—it's the pressures we let them place on us. As the comic-strip character Pogo once said: "We have met the enemy and he is us."

Every one of us has goals and dreams, and we worry about ever achieving them. We worry about secrets we have that might be found out. We try to display our good qualities and correct our character defects. We also have flaws we try to hide from the world—and sometimes from ourselves. This leads to a lot of conflict, tension and frustration—in short, stress.

Many people have low self-esteem. They may appear successful to the world, but deep inside they're somehow convinced that they're failures.

Our everyday lives also hold a variety of fears—loss of a job, rocky relationships, money troubles, criminal attack, polluted air. The list can be unending. Stress makes it even worse, since fear is a natural and immediate psychological response to stress.

Some people are more likely to suffer from chronic stress because they inherit or develop certain personality traits that make them more prone to stress and, as a consequence, to fatigue.

LESS STRESS EQUALS MORE ENERGY

But just because you've always been stressed out doesn't mean you have to stay that way. Millions of people have learned ways to overcome other addictive and obsessive behaviors. You can do the same with stress.

Learning to cope with stress is probably the single most effective way to regain lost energy. With support from friends and family, the "walking weary" can look at themselves realistically and change who they are and how they react.

If chronic stress is the primary or a contributing cause of your fatigue, stress reduction will improve both the way you feel now and your long-term health. And even if stress has nothing to do with your tiredness, at the very least, reducing your stress levels will improve the quality of your life.

Of course life is stressful, but you don't have to let it get the best of you. Every day millions of people routinely perform activities that would intimidate many of us or stress us to exhaustion.

Think of a tightrope walker who regularly saunters along a thin cable high in the air—without a safety net. Just the thought of doing it could make many of us very nervous. Yet to the tightrope walker it's just a routine job.

Why? It is definitely dangerous. A 40-foot fall can be just as deadly to a professional tightrope walker as it is to anyone else. The difference lies in accepting the danger with confidence. That confidence usually comes with training, study, practice, experience and success.

To someone who has never done this trick, only the dangers are apparent. For a professional it's as easy as walking across the driveway.

Let's take another example. Do you remember the first time you drove a car in traffic and how nervous you were?

When you took your driver's test you had the training. Now that same training is backed up by years of experience. Your confidence has grown with your experience.

If stress is a major problem, you must learn how to keep the stress-causing elements of your life from getting to you. But to do that, you have to determine what causes your stress. Is it part of your job, your lifestyle, your relationships or your attitude toward life, yourself and other people?

GIANT STEPS TOWARD STRESS REDUCTION

Before you can reduce your stress level, you have to identify the source of that stress and how it affects your life. To do that, you must get to know yourself well.

Individuals react in different ways, so an activity that reduces stress for one person may increase it for another. For example, suppose you decide to take up running. You do it because running makes you feel better physically, takes your mind off your problems and helps you recapture the childhood joy of running free. Under such circumstances, running will probably lower your stress levels and improve your physical health. On the other hand, if you obsess about running, turn it into a job, become overly competitive, set unrealistic goals for yourself and then hate yourself for not meeting them, running will just *add* to your stress.

So when you look for a way to reduce stress, look for the one that will work for *you.* That's why you need to know who you are.

Stress results from your unique reaction to certain things that touch your life. It starts inside your head, so that's where you begin the search for your true self. Start by taking a close, objective look at yourself. You can afford to be honest, since no one but you will ever know what you see, unless you choose to tell.

Are you scared of losing your job or the love of your family? Do you fear dogs, crowds or meeting new people? Do you agonize over mistakes or other people's opinions of you? Are you afraid of looking foolish?

Everyone has fears, so be honest with yourself. We don't always recognize them because they are cleverly hidden behind some logical thought process. You might want to earn more money

WHAT CHRONIC STRESS DOES TO YOUR HEALTH

Chronic stress is a co-conspirator with disease in a movement to wreck your health. Adrenaline and certain other chemicals called into play by stress increase heart rate and blood pressure. This puts a strain on the blood vessels, inviting high blood pressure and hardening of the arteries. These "stress chemicals" also increase the amount of fatty acids in the blood, contributing to atherosclerosis and heart attacks. To further complicate matters, stress is one of the main reasons people say they smoke—in itself a major cause of high blood pressure and heart attacks.

Even though studies done over the past 20 years show that stress has the greatest impact on the heart and blood vessels, the damage doesn't stop there. Over time stress chemicals impair the immune system's ability to fight infections. This doesn't mean that everyone suffering from chronic stress will develop serious infections. But researchers have found lower levels of T-lymphocytes, key "soldiers" in your body's defense against illness. Stress also results in more frequent, more severe and longer-lasting colds and infections.

Some researchers think the effect of stress on the immune system is what links chronic stress to cancer and certain types of tumors. This has yet to be proven, but convincing clues keep researchers working on it. According to one theory, stress does not actually cause cancer, but it makes the immune system more vulnerable and less able to respond. That allows cancer to take hold more readily. The effect chronic stress has on the immune system may also explain why people who suffer from stress are more prone to arthritis and Graves' disease (an overactive thyroid gland).

Back and neck pain, migraines and stress headaches are also linked to chronic stress, which maintains high tension levels in our muscles.

Stress also opens the airways so more oxygen can get into the lungs to meet the immediate increase in energy demand. But with chronic stress this response burns out and actually causes air passages to shrink. This leads to asthma.

Stress also forces the body to produce more stomach acid, leading to ulcers.

Finally, a great deal of evidence shows that being in a state of chronic stress makes a person more accident-prone. And of course, when your health is compromised in any of these various ways, you feel weary.

at your job, for example, but you hesitate to apply for a higher position because of the fear of not excelling at new responsibilities. So you suffer in silence—and your self-esteem suffers as well. Or you hate it when your mother spoils your children, but you seethe inside rather than speaking up because you're afraid of what she might say.

The truth is that we experience more stress when we *don't* confront our fears. It's a lot like being a kid in bed with the lights out, convinced that there's a monster in the room. You can hear it moving around! It's there! The longer you hide under the covers, the bigger and more terrible the monster grows in your imagination. But when you finally work up the courage to come out of hiding and turn on the lights, the source of your worry turns out to be the family cat, or the shadow of a toy, or a branch brushing against your bedroom window.

Fears take on more substance in the dark. Try shining a light on some of yours. You'll find them much easier to face.

Facing your fears and conquering them does wonders for your self-esteem. But until you admit to having some fears, you can neither face nor conquer them.

Everybody has a harrowing story or two to tell about the agony stress has put them through. Here is a guide to avoiding a few of the many types of stressful situations that can trap anyone. The point to remember is that you usually have a choice about letting yourself get trapped in the first place. And even when you can't avoid the problem, you can choose how you react to it—with stress, or without.

Declare self-ownership. Are you overwhelmed by demands placed upon you by others? Your boss? Spouse? Children? Friends? Co-workers? Advocates of good causes? People you barely know? Do you go through your days feeling that everyone has a right to run your life except you? If the answer to any of the above is yes, ask yourself why.

Some people place themselves in a position where they have too much to answer for because they crave responsibility. It makes them feel important. Being needed provides purpose in life for some people. It justifies their existence and gives them an identity. But they become so deeply involved with the fortunes of others that they forget about themselves. People pleasers are those who are afraid that if they ever say no to a request, they'll lose all their friends. In reality that rarely happens.

People pleasers often find themselves feeling emotionally and physically spent. Perhaps you're one of them. Are the demands placed on you appropriate for just one person? Have you said no to an unreasonable or inconvenient request during the past week, or even the past month? Did it make you uncomfortable to do so? Work at giving yourself permission to choose which sacrifices of time and effort you will make. Don't sign up for unnecessary stress.

Communicate clearly. As we saw earlier, stress is a form of mental labor. We must list personal relationships high among the most energy-intensive jobs we have in life. These relationships are formed and maintained by communication. And failure to communicate clearly results in anxiety, worry, fear and doubt, especially for a person who tends to assume the worst. "What does he think?" "What will she say?" "Did she mean . . . ?" "Do they understand that meant . . . ?"

This requires a lot of energy and can be tiring. Be honest and clear, and expect the same of others. If they are not forthcoming, let it be their problem. When you are in doubt, ask people what they really mean. Then take their words at face value. If they claim later that you didn't understand what they "really meant," remind them of those words. If they persist in playing games, let them play alone. Refuse to be drawn into a relationship based on the need to figure out hidden meanings and obscure signals. Unless you are dealing with a mind reader, expecting someone to "know" what you are thinking can only lead to disappointment and resentment.

Saying, "If he really loved me, he'd know what I want" or "If she really cared, she'd understand what I really mean" is an exercise in futility (and yes, a waste of energy).

Honesty requires admitting mistakes. Suppose you miss a lunch meeting with a friend—you just plain forget. The simplest thing is to call and apologize by admitting that it slipped your mind. It may be embarrassing, but we all know such things happen, and no one has ever died from embarrassment.

A real friend will accept your explanation. No anxiety. No stress. You might get teased about your sievelike memory, but you'll probably feel you deserve it. An awkward situation has turned into fun instead of emotional anguish.

But suppose you decide to lie—to protect your ego and try to avoid the appearance of fallibility by making up a story about some crisis you had to attend to. You may never know if your friend really believed you or was merely being polite. But you do worry. Also, you have to remember the lie in case the subject comes up two weeks later.

The phrase "Honesty is the best policy" is a cliché—and for a good reason. In the long run, it avoids a lot of unnecessary stress.

Don't be drawn into a no-win situation. Anyone caught in a double bind or no-win situation is lost. You have two choices, and both are bad. So naturally, double binds create stress. For example, imagine that you have two friends who are fighting and each of them asks you to agree that the other is wrong. What do you do? The intelligent response is to tell both friends that you will not take sides. You hope they can work it out. But you will still be a friend to both, whatever the outcome.

That sounds easy, but it isn't, especially when the parties pressure you to get involved in the argument. Double binds make us feel completely helpless, impotent. Whatever we do will be wrong or lead to more problems. We throw up our hands; our stress levels rise.

Don't let yourself be dragged into a losing proposition. Don't let yourself become an emotional hostage.

If you learn that your friendship hangs on agreeing with one or the other, it's not much of a friendship. And if they end it, that's their decision and their problem.

Stay out of double binds. Getting involved can only lead to pain, embarrassment and stress. If you tell either or both friends you're on their side, you have the short-term gain of being happy. You also suffer the long-term pain of being in the middle of the fight. In summary: Short-term gain, long-term pain.

If, on the other hand, you stay out of the fight, you may be uncomfortable, feeling the need to help your two friends solve the problem. But you force yourself to stay out of their business. Your stress is reduced in the long run. You end up with short-term pain, long-term gain.

Don't identify yourself with your job. Work is a major cause of both stress and emotional burnout: high-pressure jobs, deadlines, demanding bosses, angry clients, impatient customers, poor working conditions, low pay and misunderstandings with co-workers. We come home from work late at night exhausted, but that's not our fault, we say—it's the stress of the job. Is it really?

Actually there are two kinds of work-related stress: true and phony. The latter is a product of burying yourself in work and creating job stress in order to avoid or deny some other problem or situation.

Workaholics are the best example of this. They blame the stress on their demanding work, when, in fact, it is an excuse to avoid dealing with a problem at home. It is rarely because they need more money. People who work extra hard for long hours, creating high stress levels, rarely earn much more than those working a regular shift.

In earlier chapters we noted the need for a sense of fulfillment and excitement about our work, career or goals. Work can be important in creating a healthy sense of self-worth if it is fun, fulfilling and energizing. Professional effort is healthy, and its role in your life should be positive, with goals that go beyond a regular paycheck and steady work. Fulfilling these goals adds to the sense of healthy excitement and vitality in your life.

But too few jobs provide all of that. Therefore, so many people find fulfillment and satisfy their "professional striving" through involvement with joblike activities that include community theater, sports, social or church work, hobbies and fraternal or professional associations. That's fine. The important thing is to find a sense of self-worth. Where you get it isn't important. But you should know that the same problems, pressures and attitudes that can cause stress on a job can also cause it in other activities.

So examine your job and any joblike activities you engage in. Do they cause unnecessary stress? Are you doing the work of two people? Are you moving in the right direction or going the wrong way? Do you have a life outside the office? If not, you certainly should.

Discuss these matters openly with your boss or with others you report to or work with. They will respect you for having a sense of purpose and direction because they know it can be good for the entire operation.

But what if that doesn't work? Then you have two choices: Change your job or activities—or change your attitude. We'll look at some concrete techniques for changing attitude in the next chapter.

The main thing to remember is that no matter how dedicated you are to your job, at some point it's healthy to walk away, emotionally and physically.

Be choosy about how you spend your leisure. Stressors of all kinds surround us, and often they're disguised as sources of fun, like movies, computer games and television programs. They all take their toll in energy.

TV is just one example. How do you feel after watching yet another show about battered wives, abused children, people being blown up, terrible monsters, terrorists or politics? *That's* entertainment?

Do you really need to watch such stories on TV or at the movies? Do you really need to read a horror tale or a thriller just before trying to wind down for the night? Is the newspaper or the 11 o'clock news a calming influence when you're about to turn off the light? Can you relax while spending an hour on a computer game that involves blowing up buildings, beating up terrorists, tracking down a master criminal or shooting down jet planes? Try something soothing for a change.

As we get older, we're more likely to suffer from stress. That's because aging tends to make people more fixed in their ways, less flexible intellectually. It's harder for them to face new demands and changes.

It doesn't have to be that way. While you do have to get older, nothing says that you must become inflexible. You can work at staying open to new experiences, new ways of doing things and new ideas. Not only will you avoid getting stuck in the past, you'll learn to live in the present—and enjoy it.

CHAPTER

11

Stress Busters

You're never really stuck with stress. There are dozens of simple, practical and effective methods you can use to lower stress levels so you can have the energetic and fulfilling life you yearn for. Many of these aids were proven effective in scientific tests; others demonstrated their worth in practice among generations of people who found them effective.

Regardless of the cause of your fatigue, stress makes it worse. And simply getting rid of that stress turns things around by releasing bursts of new energy.

Here are 25 techniques you can use to cast off the burden of fatigue by cutting stress. Some will work better for you than others because stress reduction, like stress itself, is very personal. When you find those that do the trick for you, make them a regular part of your life.

At the end of this chapter you will find 15 "quick fixes" to use when you need to be calm and patient—right now!

GET PHYSICAL

Three of the best ways to reduce stress and regain lost energy are exercise, exercise and exercise, since physical activity lets the mind relax. Fatigue from exercise is muscle fatigue, not brain fatigue. After you finish working out, that fatigue is quickly replaced by vitality and feelings of accomplishment. More than that, exercise does as much for your body and overall physical health and well-being as it does for your stress.

The only time exercise won't help is when fatigue and stress stem from a medical problem (a severe heart condition, for example) that could be aggravated by physical exertion. But in such a case you should be under your doctor's care anyway. Ask the doctor if exercise is appropriate in your personal situation.

Popular options include aerobics at a health club or gym, home-based exercise with special equipment, a sport like jogging or tennis and so forth. The type of exercise you choose doesn't really matter, provided you do it regularly. Make it a habit.

Try walking while making up your mind. You might want to start out with a one-mile walk before breakfast or after dinner. By the time you've decided, you might be up to three miles a day. And even though a sidewalk stroll may lack the pizzazz of an upbeat aerobics class, it has these advantages: It is always available, it requires little equipment and there's no fee, plus you never have to call ahead to make a reservation.

Best of all, a walking program is unlikely to turn into yet another source of stress. (You certainly don't need that! Stress is what got you into the shape you're in.) You're not competing to set a world record or trying to beat 50 other walkers. Besides, in terms of stress relief, walking a slow mile every day is better than a gung ho game of racquetball once a month.

As an added plus, if you pick interesting places to walk and are joined by a good friend, you soon forget that you're exercising. You're having *fun.*

SET GOALS YOU CAN FOCUS ON

Set priorities in your life. Many people feel stressed because they don't know what they want to do or even what they *can* do. They feel useless and unfocused, and they see their life as a waste.

What are your goals? What comes first in your life, then second, and what comes after that? Think in terms of both long-term and short-term goals, personal aims as well as professional ambitions.

THE CASE OF THE COMPULSIVE RUNNER

Bob was a 40-year-old stressed-out executive, and the pressure was finally getting to him. Not only was he constantly anxious, but he was tired all the time. Bob knew he had to do something, but what?

He'd been an athlete in school and was still slim and in fairly good shape. So he decided to exercise to reduce his stress. He'd start running. But his running program was designed to do more than reduce stress. He had another goal: He was determined to run around the park trail at least five minutes faster than the half hour it took most people to do it. The task was a daunting one.

Bob pursued his running goal the same way he pursued goals at work–with dedication, determination, singleness of purpose and a total disregard for what it did to him.

Instead of reducing his stress levels and helping him get back his lost energy, Bob's running program *added* to his stress and fatigue.

He finally realized what he was doing to himself and switched from beat-the-clock running to relaxed jogging. Bob also took more time off from work and stopped looking at life as if it were a competitive sport. When he did, he regained his lost energy and began enjoying life again.

Remember that your personal life is not limited to your relationships. If you have a mate, of course that relationship is important; if you are a parent, being a good one is important, too. But so is achieving personal goals that have nothing to do with your family—going back to school, volunteering for community work, reading more books and so forth. (By the way, having fun and enjoying life are also worthwhile goals.) Live up to the demands of your important aim.

Realizing those goals will give you far more fulfillment than lesser accomplishments. Also, it's not as likely that you'll get stressed out when you can't or don't want to do something unimportant to you or something that interferes with what is important to you. Don't let unnecessary stresses run you down and destroy your attempts at success in the things that count for you.

One final point: You are allowed to change your goals. So don't be afraid to change your mind if a goal you set today no longer seems appealing or practical six months from now.

KEEP A STRESS DIARY

Make a daily record of things you do that cause you stress by answering the following questions. You needn't give long answers; just write enough to jog your memory later.

1. What was the demand or situation that caused stress?
2. Why did you do it? Was it a duty or obligation, an order, something expected of you? Did you do it out of love, to impress someone, because no one else would? Did you realize what you were getting into when you agreed to do it? If you don't know why you did it, write that down.
3. Was the stress escalated or diminished as the situation unfolded?
4. Did you experience the same or similar stress previously, with either greater or less intensity, and what, if anything, made it different this time?
5. What did you feel—a sense of accomplishment, or wasted time and effort—when you finished?
6. Did the stress continue after you completed the task, and if so, how long?
7. How did the stress affect the rest of your day?
8. Was the job worth the stress?
9. Was the stress really necessary?
10. Would you do the activity again, given a choice?

Keep the diary for a typical week, then study it for patterns. Maybe the stress is tied, not to what you do, but rather to the conditions under which you do it or who's involved.

Go through your diary and mark all those things that were stressful and totally unnecessary. You will be surprised at how many stresses you can easily eliminate once you become aware of them.

If you are seeing a therapist, take your diary along to your next session, so you can discuss what you discovered. Getting an impartial second opinion can be a great help. (Reviewing your stress diary with a spouse, parent or someone else who is emotionally involved with you doesn't count as an impartial opinion. It might even be dangerous to your stress levels.)

FACE STRESS WITH STRENGTH

No life is completely stress free. You cannot avoid certain stressful situations. Some arise out of emergencies. Others are the inevitable ones you can see coming—like college tuition or balding—and have plenty of time to dread.

You have a limited amount of energy. In stressful situations, concentrate that energy where it will do the most good. Let's look at three examples.

1. You're home on a Sunday morning and your young daughter falls and breaks her arm. You have to get her to the hospital—either you call an ambulance, drive her yourself or get someone else to drive you both.

   You'll probably spend hours in the emergency room dealing with a terrified child and her pain. You'll be frightened and concerned. You'll also have to handle the waiting and the paperwork, plus receptionists, doctors and nurses.

   The plans you made for the day have to be changed. People will have to be called, schedules rearranged. But your child needs you. That's what parenthood is all about.
2. You love your job, and one of its main advantages for you is that you don't have to travel. Due to a new merger, however, you are required to make a long plane trip. You hate to fly. But this trip is very important to your career—a career that you find satisfying, enjoyable and profitable.

   After weighing the alternatives, you decide that you will make the trip. You aren't happy about it, but you will do it.
3. You are moving into a new house in three weeks. There is no such thing as a stress-free move. In terms of stress, many experts say that moving ranks right up there with getting a new job or losing a loved one.

When such a situation is unavoidable, meet the stress firmly and effectively. Rather than becoming rattled, focus on what you have to do, think about why you are doing it, and look forward to its ending. Don't let yourself get caught up in less important matters that only add unnecessary stress.

If you and your spouse are at the hospital with an injured child, for example, you may have other children at home who need care. Don't worry about cooking dinner for them or making sure they take their baths and get to bed on time; just make sure someone is there to take care of them. Then, once you've given instructions to the caregiver, forget about it and concentrate on the emergency at hand.

If you have to fly even though you absolutely hate it, make the trip as easy on yourself as possible. Have a friend or associate drive you to the airport or take an airport limo, and hire a skycap to take care of your luggage. That minimizes the stress involved in getting to the airport, parking and checking your luggage.

Investigate ways to overcome your fear of flying—try a therapy group or a class. (Some companies will even pick up the tab.) To track down possible resources for help, call one of the major airlines.

If you have to move, accept the fact that there is no way to do it without stress. But you can reduce that stress if you plan ahead, cut down on other commitments, pack in advance and ask friends to help out.

In other words, try to anticipate stressful situations and take steps ahead of time to reduce the stress.

After getting through a stressful situation you will probably feel better about yourself. You're entitled. After all, you did something you didn't want to do, something that frightened you.

In one sense stress can be seen as fear itself, and fear, when confronted directly, usually turns out to be unfounded.

When you avoid unnecessary complications and focus on dealing with the single problem at hand, the situation loses some of its power to frighten you. *If* there is a next time, you'll be even better prepared.

ACCEPT LIMITATIONS

In the preceding chapter you were advised to get to know yourself better. Now it's time to look at your abilities and limitations. You know what they are. In fact, you've probably been fighting, denying or hiding behind many of them for years. That is as tiring as it is stressful.

The key point here is a simple one: Limitations are not failures. For example, a man who is 5 feet tall can't expect to make it in professional basketball, and a woman who is 6 feet tall can't hope for a career as a jockey. That doesn't mean that short men can't play basketball or that tall women can't ride horses. They can and do—to the best of their abilities. But in terms of doing it as a career, well, every job has its requirements. So do many hobbies.

Don't hide behind your limitations; accept them and concentrate on what you can do. Maybe you can't be the best, but that doesn't mean you can't be very good.

No one, not even you, can do everything perfectly. Accept that. Also accept the fact that other people have limitations, too. Expecting the near impossible from others, or setting too-high expectations, can let you down again and again.

LIVE YOUR OWN LIFE

Too many of us believe that our stress would disappear if only someone else in our life would shape up. But that's not true.

Your life doesn't really depend on someone else's actions or moods. You can be happy and stress free if you decide to live your own life and not wait for someone else to change.

The only person you can change is yourself. Work on that, and you'll feel more fulfilled and less stressed than if you were to focus on someone else's actions as the key to your happiness.

CALL TIME-OUT

Reserve a block of time every day just for yourself. Don't let anything short of an emergency interfere with it. And be careful what you call an emergency. Don't answer the telephone. Don't let people know where you are. Don't respond when someone calls. You are entitled to time by yourself, so take it.

Start out with 15 minutes a day, until you get used to the idea. (If you start off with an hour you just might panic, feel guilty or get bored.) After a week or so, stretch it to a half hour or an hour. You decide how much time you want and when to take it—morning coffee break, after lunch, early evening.

Don't let anyone—not even your spouse or children or co-workers—talk you out of taking that time-out or into "sharing" it with them. This is your time. Tell the others to take time off for themselves and that you'll see them after the session.

Use the time any way you wish, but make it stress free. Read a magazine; lie down; take a walk in the park.

Perhaps you've always wanted to try writing poetry or painting or learning how to juggle. This is a good time to do it—provided you don't take it too seriously. If you decide to write or paint, be prepared to throw out the first efforts. If you want to learn how to juggle, don't be disappointed if you drop the balls often at first. As long as you don't expect to be perfect, there will be no pressure.

You can count on a million interruptions during the first weeks, but don't give in. Eventually stress will begin to fade and you'll look forward to your private time with the same anticipation you feel for meeting an old friend.

The people at work and those you live with might question you about these periods alone, even accuse you of being irresponsible and wasting time. On the contrary; reducing your stress levels helps you live up to your responsibilities. You become stronger, more vital and more responsible.

PUT AWAY YOUR WATCH

Do you really need a watch? There are clocks in cars, in offices, on the kitchen stove, on computers, on fax machines, in store windows and outside of banks and office buildings. Radio stations announce the time frequently. In fact, it's hard to go anywhere without being aware of what time it is.

If you wear a watch because you're always checking it to stay on schedule, you're likely to get more and more stressed out because the time may be passing too slowly or too quickly to suit you.

Leave your watch at home for a week. If you have to know what time it is, ask one of those who wear a watch. Let *them* obsess about how quickly or slowly the time passes.

Knowing the exact time doesn't make you more efficient, smarter, richer or calmer. All it does is tempt you to think of it and worry.

TAKE A MENTAL HEALTH DAY

Everyone is entitled to take sick days, so why not take a day off as a mental health day? Stress causes more trouble than all the cases of colds and flu combined. When you are stressed, you need to take time to recover from it—maybe a day away from work or a day away from your family.

But don't rush into it. After you become used to the idea of taking some time out for yourself every day and being nice to yourself in small doses, and once you begin to see the benefits, you'll look forward to having a whole day to yourself.

Use your day off for an activity you know you'll enjoy or to do something you've always wanted to try. The only criterion is that it must be fun for you.

LEARN TO SAY NO

It's amazing how often we walk into a stressful situation with our eyes open, our fists clenched and our mouths clamped shut to prevent us from screaming. Sometimes we even pack up the kids and take them along so they can be stressed out, too.

Family gatherings, especially around the holidays, can be filled with stress. But many of us feel we have to attend, no matter how painful or embarrassing we expect the affair to be. Besides, this time might be different, even though these parties have been miserable for the last 5 or 10 or 50 times.

What would people think if you didn't show up, or if you attended but left early? How would it look if you flew in to your hometown and then stayed at a hotel to avoid being surrounded by family 24 hours a day?

The folks might think you figured out how to take care of yourself. They might even respect your stand in declining to do something hurtful to you.

It's true that some families are a major source of stress to certain members, but there are plenty of other occasions of psychological anguish. For example, we often attend social gatherings, parties, business functions and other affairs that we dread, simply because we're convinced we "have to."

On another level, we sometimes accept jobs, promotions or other "marvelous opportunities" we know we will hate out of a sense of obligation—and fear that we might never get another chance. And again: "What would people think?" Does it matter? Your obligation is to guard your stress level so you can actually feel alive instead of merely existing.

If you really don't want to do something, say so.

Of course, there are some stressful situations you cannot say no to, but not nearly as many as you might think. Learn to decipher the difference between "I have to do this because there is no choice" and "I do not have to do this because I do have choices."

Learn to stand up for yourself and take care of yourself by saying no. The stress you save will be your own.

LAUGH LOUD AND OFTEN

One of the most effective and enjoyable stress relievers in the world is laughter. There is nothing like a funny movie, book or comedian, a friend with a wonderful sense of humor or just plain being silly to ease any tension you feel. Many people invest in games and toys for that very reason. Piling building blocks to create the tallest tower you can and then knocking it down with a toy truck as toddlers do could be your ticket to lightening up.

Take time to joke and relax. Learn to laugh at yourself. Stress levels go down when you refuse to take yourself too seriously.

Laughter can also do wonders for relationships. Actress Joanne Woodward, when asked why she had stayed married to Paul Newman for so many years, replied simply: "He makes me laugh."

The plus factor is that laughter does not require a visit to the doctor for a prescription, a nurse to administer it or an insurance company to pay for it.

SET REALISTIC DEADLINES

There are only 24 hours in a day, and most of those hours are earmarked for rest and relaxation. You have things that must get done, so you do have to manage your time effectively. But *you* manage the time; don't let the time manage you.

Be flexible. Avoid committing to time limits unless you're sure the job can be done properly in that time.

The stress involved with accomplishing something within a tight deadline can be enormous. It might lead to overwork, sleeplessness, anger, frustration and resentment.

It's a common mistake for people to set impossible time limits for themselves—and others—and to work under the pressure such deadlines impose. They do it again and again, never giving themselves enough time to do the job properly or to rest up for the next one. Often the result is both exhaustion and failure.

One standard lament is that there is never enough time to get a job done right, yet there's always enough time to do it all over again when it comes out wrong. If you allot the necessary time at the outset, you won't need more time to redo it later.

KEEP YOUR COOL

You have two arms, two legs, two eyes, two ears—but only one brain. That means you can concentrate on only one thing at a time. If you try to do more, you're asking for trouble, frustration and stress.

Here's an example. Dinner is on the stove, the baby is crying, the phone rings, the pot boils over and the four-year-old falls onto a sharp table corner—all at the same time.

Obviously, you can't take care of everything all at once. The only way to get through this is to decide what has to be done first, and do it. Then tackle the next thing, and so on.

There are times when your life does get overloaded unavoidably. But overloading deliberately is unwise and dangerous for your mental health.

DUMP THE CAFFEINE

Since the fatigue-related effects of caffeine are covered in chapter 17, let's consider only its addictive properties. If you are addicted to caffeine, quitting cold turkey will be hard. It can cause severe headaches for a week or so. However, if you wean yourself by drinking a half-and-half mixture of regular coffee and decaf, the odds are that you won't have any problems. Over a couple of weeks reduce the amount of regular. Soon you will be able to drink straight decaf. The difference will be apparent: less jitters, less anxiety and less fatigue. Surely you can get used to that.

CHOOSE SNACKS CAREFULLY

What you eat is important to your stress level. Increased intake of fruits and vegetables not only encourages better health, it acts to reduce stress as well. These foods provide the kind of high-quality sustenance your body needs to survive and thrive.

Some people find they react to eating rich or sugary snacks or dessert foods by experiencing radical mood swings that might include feelings of lethargy and depression. They sometimes compare it to a hangover without the liquor. If this description seems to fit you, consult your doctor. If you have trouble giving up these foods, or if you turn to food for stress relief, look for support in therapy or self-help groups, such as Overeaters Anonymous.

DECIDE NOT TO DECIDE—FOR NOW

Put off important decisions until after a good night's sleep. You can't count on having a dream that tells you what to do, but you should wake up refreshed and stress free so you can figure out the best course of action.

Few major decisions have to be made on the spot—no matter what you hear from co-workers, salespeople, lawyers, family or anyone else. A decision important enough to cause stress deserves calm and pressure-free consideration. Sleeping on a problem prevents you from making a decision in haste. You become more confident, levelheaded and stress free.

NIP STRESS BEFORE IT NIPS YOU

After a period of stress has wiped you out, leaving you totally exhausted, you can sometimes remember a warning from your body before the stress hit. In the preceding chapter we saw the face of stress and how the body reacts to it—rapid heartbeat, clammy skin, sweaty palms, dry mouth, a burst of energy, increased alertness and so forth. Learn to recognize these hints early. When you detect them, ask yourself if this stress is necessary.

If you are driving along an unfamiliar road at night in the middle of a blinding rainstorm, the answer is probably yes. If you are at home watching a horror movie on TV and hoping to get right to sleep as soon as it is over, you know the answer.

CONSIDER MEDITATION

Meditation is probably the best technique to relax tensions, lower stress and reduce fatigue. It is an art and a skill that is acquired with practice. Meditation can eliminate stress completely in most people. But discipline and determination are required to learn its effective application.

For some, meditation is an end in itself. Others couple it with prayer or use it to achieve a more rewarding spiritual life.

To be effective, meditation must be taken seriously and planned for. You might make it part of that daily time-out we discussed earlier or set aside a specific meditation time. If you are constantly interrupted or distracted, your meditation will not be effective.

Even though it is very easy, relaxing and pleasurable once you get the hang of it, meditation is not for everyone. In some cases, people respond to it negatively because of common misconceptions. Meditation is not a fad. It is not a turbaned guru sitting in the lotus position on a mountaintop, striving for nirvana. It does not require a special robe, incense, chanting or Eastern music. One dictionary defines *meditation* simply as "continued or extended thought, contemplation or reflection."

And what do you contemplate? How about nature, yourself and your relationship with a higher power—God, Jesus, Buddha, Allah, the Great Spirit, the cosmic whole? The choice is yours. By its very nature, meditation is one of the most private acts you will ever engage in. You reduce the world to you and a single subject, eliminating all thoughts or ideas that interfere with that concept.

There are many different methods of meditation. Read "Meditation for Beginners" on page 126 for a common, simple method used by many people.

Meditation needs to be disciplined and regular—perhaps 15 minutes or a half hour a day, maybe twice a day. Once it has become a part of your life, you can induce a stress-reducing meditation in just a few minutes. Unlike waking from a nap, foggy and groping for a cup of coffee, you will emerge relaxed and refreshed.

Sometimes meditation leads to a desire to help others. Selflessness is clearly effective in reducing stress. You get involved with someone else's life and problems, and in concentrating on them, you forget yourself and your own problems.

Editor's Note: If you are being treated for depression, consult your doctor or therapist before attempting meditation on your own.

IMAGINE YOU CAN DO IT

Positive imagery is a form of meditation in which thoughts are directed toward creating a positive mental attitude. Such images and experiences are brought to the surface and looked at. It is like having a pleasant dream where the effects remain with you even after you have awakened.

Positive imagery is a form of autohypnosis, a meditative trance that you induce and you control. It can be used in many ways.

For example, if you fear flying, spend time imagining yourself in a plane—safe, warm, carefree and comfortable.

MEDITATION FOR BEGINNERS

Create a time and place where no disruption will occur. Turn on the answering machine or take the phone off the hook. Isolate yourself.

Get comfortable: Loosen your belt, take off your shoes, open your collar, take off your jacket. But don't get so comfortable that you will fall asleep.

- Sit on the floor with cushions supporting your lower back, or sit in a comfortable but firm chair with your feet flat on the floor.
- Close your eyes and start to relax each muscle group in your body, one by one. Normal thought processes continue, but instead of being directed toward the day's stresses, they are directed to relaxation.
- Start at the toes and work up. Relax everything. Contract the muscles in your toes, and then relax them. Do the same with your ankles, calf muscles, knees and so on, all the way up to your scalp. At first this is quite difficult, and it takes some time and practice. You might even feel foolish. That's just one of the reasons you should do it while you are alone.
- Don't worry if you have problems. By the time you relax your face, you may notice that your legs are tense again. Don't expect to do it perfectly. Just work on getting better every time. With practice and repetition, this relaxation occurs quite quickly. The body relaxes but the mind stays alert—not sleepy, alert.
- Focus your thoughts on a single subject—maybe on a sunset, a butterfly, a work of art, the ocean, the desert, your

Positive imagery can also help prepare you for an event, a meeting, even a test. Let's say you are going to be making an important presentation. Visualize going through it: You stand there before the group, organized and in control. You know what you will say, and you say it well. You run through the questions that will be raised, and when they are, you have the answers. You resolve difficulties before they can turn into problems. You do a great job.

This way, when you actually give that presentation, you will already have done it in your head. You'll know what to expect, so you'll experience less stress.

heartbeat, maybe even on God. See it in your mind's eye. You aren't trying to figure anything out. You are just there, relaxed and contemplative.

Let's say you contemplate a sunset over the ocean. Even though you're not there, you experience it. You see the red-orange light of the sun reflected off the water, hear the seabirds call, smell the ocean, taste the salt air, feel the sandy beach against your bare feet, shiver a bit as the cool wind fans your face.

- Other thoughts will come up. Don't fight them. If you remember that the car needs a new muffler, just say, "That's right . . . " and let the thought go. Don't think about where you're going to take the car to be fixed, how you're going to pay for it, the warranty on the old muffler or anything else. Yes, the car needs a new muffler—but not this instant. Next you may start to think about an argument you had the night before. Don't dwell on it, just let it go.
- Look at these thoughts like trains. You can hop on and get carried away, or let them go on down the track without you. In many ways it's like watching yourself dream. Most thoughts come in the front door, a few enter from side doors, and occasionally one slips in the back door. The back-door thoughts are the really interesting ones.
- Watch the thoughts and separate yourself from thinking them. Don't try to direct them, discover anything or strive for anything. Just watch and let the thoughts flow.
- Eventually the random thoughts will stop, and you'll be able to really enjoy the sunset. And when you are finished you'll find that you've had 15 or 30 stress-free minutes.

This method is very effective, but it also requires discipline and consistency.

LOOK INTO BIOFEEDBACK

In biofeedback you learn to understand how your body responds to the emotional state you are in. We already saw that stress changes your heartbeat, blood chemistry, brain waves, muscle tension and so on. Biofeedback machines measure these changes and let you see or hear the results. With this information, you can learn how to control your physical and emotional state.

Let's say, for example, that you are hyperventilating. You can look at the machine's dials and see what that condition does to your heartbeat, brain waves, muscle tension and the like. As you slow your breathing, you can see the changes in your readings. Seeing the immediate and actual effects of your actions—and thoughts—helps you learn what to do to correct them. This can be an aid to meditation and relaxation.

There are many forms of biofeedback. It has become an accepted medical therapy for many conditions, including stress, insomnia, high blood pressure, migraine headaches and seizure disorders. Your doctor or local hospital can provide more information about biofeedback.

CONSIDER COUNSELING

You don't have to be "crazy" to consult a psychiatrist or a counselor. In fact, it could be one way for you to avoid going crazy!

Counseling is designed to help you to know yourself better. That makes it easier to resolve your fears and anxieties and overcome stress. One reason stress leads to fatigue is that, for some, the battle against fear and anxiety seems hopeless. They think they might as well give up, quit, spend the rest of their life in bed.

A trustworthy, experienced counselor or therapist can help you find ways to win your battles. Overcoming a personal problem will give you a great feeling of accomplishment. Your mind and body will want to celebrate—and you'll actually have the energy to do so.

Chronic fatigue is like a stuffy room filled with stale cigarette smoke. We put up with it because we are in the room and do not know how to change the air. With personal growth and self-knowledge, windows are opened and the breeze that blows through clears the air.

GET A PET

If you don't have the means or the inclination to seek counseling, friendly, low-maintenance pets—like a cat or a pair of goldfish—might take the edge off stress. Studies have shown that stroking a pet for a few minutes can lower blood pressure. And grousing to your goldfish averts the bad feeling that can come from complaining to friends or family when you come home from work feeling out of sorts.

PASS UP PILLS

Tranquilizers do reduce stress. If you're suitably drugged, you can go through anything without getting stressed—a death in the family, getting fired, being evicted, anything. Doctors prescribe tranquilizers because they work, and they work fast.

But tranquilizers handle stress the way that wallpaper handles a man-sized hole in the outside wall of a skyscraper. It hides the problem but doesn't solve it; you never know when someone will fall through the hole and die.

Second, tranquilizers are addictive. When you eventually come off the medication, your life problems are right in front of you again, perhaps even worse than before. The level of stress will be greater as well. Also, you will have to go through withdrawal, an uncomfortable period that's often far worse than whatever stress the pills were originally prescribed for.

Used cautiously and for short periods, tranquilizers can be an aid to other forms of stress reduction. They are helpful for extreme life crises such as the death of a loved one, or when used in conjunction with psychological therapy, and in some types of sleep disorders. And they can be a useful tool in an overall treatment plan for phobias and panic attacks. But when chronic fatigue is due to stress, the problem is not the fatigue you feel but the stress that causes or contributes to it. You don't cure stress by covering it up.

DON'T STAY ANGRY

Anger may get your heart pumping, but not in the beneficial way that aerobic exercise does. Like stress, anger is a perfectly natural emotion. But also like stress, chronic anger can kill you, or at least leave you shaken and drained.

You cannot prevent yourself from ever getting angry. But you can control the emotion and reduce the stress it causes.

Exercise, both competitive and noncompetitive, can be a good outlet for anger and aggression. So can anything else that keeps you busy and lets you focus on something other than your anger: movies, TV, a hobby, housecleaning, yard work or any activity that gets your mind off your problem.

Sometimes you just have to talk about your anger and get it out into the open. Otherwise it can fester and grow, adding to your stress and tiredness. This is particularly true in family situations. After all, these are the people you live with.

TO BE CALM, LIVE CALMLY

You don't have to live life in the fast lane. You don't have to be surrounded by bright lights, loud noises, frantic action and hyper people. You don't have to maintain a perpetual buzz or high.

Overstimulation acts like caffeine. It creates instant energy—false energy—but is inevitably followed by more stress, tiredness or worse.

Look at yourself. Study your life. If it is a frantic, stressed-out rat race and you're not even sure why you're running—relax.

If you want to be calm, live calmly. You can do it. You do have choices in life.

15 QUICK FIXES FOR EVERYDAY AGGRAVATIONS

Meditation, keeping a stress diary, establishing priorities in your life and all the other techniques discussed so far do work. But they take time.

What can you do when you are about to explode and need relief *now?*

Here's a list of 15 quick fixes for almost-instant stress relief. Some of these work best at the office, some are best used at home, others work just fine anywhere. As you try them, you will learn which ones are most effective for you.

Remember to do one or more of these *before* you say or do anything you might later regret.

1. **Count to 10.** (In times of extreme stress, count to 20.)
2. **Go away.** Leave the room. Go to lunch. Take a walk. If you are totally stressed out, you're not doing anyone any good, especially yourself. Even if the problem is still there when you get back, you'll be better able to deal with it.
3. **Yell! Cry! Scream!** If you're suffering raw, emotional pain

and stress, make raw, emotional sounds. They don't have to make sense, just ease the pressure.

4. Pound a punching bag. A full-size punching bag weighs about 70 pounds and is built to take a lot of abuse. You can slap, punch, kick and tackle it. It doesn't fight back, and you don't have to apologize to it the next day. To save wear and tear on your hands, wear gloves. And if you don't have a punching bag, use a good-sized pillow.

5. Stretch. Stretch your whole body—neck, shoulders, arms, hands, fingers, torso, legs, ankles, toes—everything you can. Take your time. Focus on your body and what you're doing. Get the tension out of your body and you'll get it out of your mind.

6. Breathe deeply. Take deep, deep breaths. Concentrate on filling your lungs with oxygen, as much as you can hold. Hold that breath for a moment, then let it out slowly. Do it again, and again, as long as it takes to calm down.

7. Daydream. Turn your back on whatever or whoever it is that causes your stress. Sit down, close your eyes and tune out the world around you. Picture yourself where you would rather be. Enjoy being there. Consider it a mini-meditation.

8. Look away from the problem. Gaze at something far away. The closer you are, the more you have to focus and tense up your eye muscles. When you look at something in the distance, your eyes relax. And then it'll be easier to get the rest of your body to do the same.

9. Call a friend on the telephone. You're not asking that person to solve your problems, just to listen to them. Or, talk about something *besides* your problems. You'll find that talking to someone you trust who is not directly involved with the situation makes it easier for you to deal with what's bothering you.

10. Throw marshmallows. You can throw one as hard as you want at a wall. Picture windows are even better—as long as the marshmallows are soft and fresh. You're doing something physical. You hear the "Thwack!" as they hit. You see a puff of powder at impact. But nothing breaks. (This technique is especially effective in an actual fight with someone. Chances are that you'll end up laughing so hard you'll have forgotten your anger.)

11. Listen to relaxing music. Pick whatever kind you want—jazz, classical, maybe even soft rock. Heavy metal, thrash and rap are not recommended, however.

12. Go soak your body. Relax in a hot bath. Lie there and let the stress melt away. Bubble baths might help you relax, or try playing with a rubber duck.

13. Change clothes. Put on something loose and comfortable, something you feel good wearing.

14. Try self-massage. Rub your temples, your neck or whatever other muscles bunch up when you are under stress, and try to loosen them up. Concentrate on that.

15. Pray. The Serenity Prayer, an adaptation of a prayer penned by Reinhold Niebuhr in 1934, is popular with millions of people because it can and does lead to peace, calm and understanding:

> *God, grant me the serenity*
> *To accept the things I cannot change;*
> *Courage to change the things I can;*
> *And the wisdom to know the difference.*

CHAPTER

12

Depression and Other Toxic Emotions

Just as some of us react to different food additives in various ways, many of us have our own individual reactions to the equivalent emotional additives, which we might call do-it-yourself MSG—Melancholy, Shame and Guilt.

You're more likely to be successful in controlling the food additives in your diet than the emotional additives in your life. And that's not all bad. After all, a life without a wide range of ups and downs is not a life, it's merely an existence.

But we do have to establish some controls. Too much emotional energy can be more destructive than too much of a volatile food additive.

Depression, resentment, anger, hostility, grief, fear, panic, guilt, melancholy, sadness and sorrow are just some of the negative emotions we humans are subject to. They are part of life. There are times when you have every reason to be depressed, angry or sad. In fact, at those times it wouldn't be normal if you *didn't* feel that way.

Not only do such emotions affect our moods, they can affect our actions, our health and our entire attitude toward life. They can also make us very, very tired.

Understanding our emotions and learning how to deal with them can do a lot more than ease our mental state. It can also restore our energy levels and help out with certain physical problems.

The key to dealing with emotions is to face them head-on. These feelings are perfectly natural, and we can't block them, bottle them up or deny their existence without paying the price in psychological turmoil and negative physical reactions.

You can run, but you can't hide. Your emotions are part of you. Wherever you go, your emotions go, too.

A lot of people have problems dealing with this aspect of their nature. Even worse, many find real difficulty in dealing with the emotions of others. If you're one of these, you may feel compelled to tell others that they're wrong to feel the way they do. Maybe you're just trying to be helpful, but maybe you're trying to control their feelings and emotions. Do you hear yourself speaking in any of these statements? Have people said such things to you?

"You're angry? Nice people don't get angry."

"You shouldn't be sad, you should be happy. How could anyone be sad on a glorious day like today?"

"So you got laid off after 20 years, so what? Why let that ruin your day? It was only a job."

"How dare you get angry with me! I'm your mother."

"What—still not over the funeral? That was six months ago. It's time to cheer up and face the world. You should start dating again."

"You're too big to cry. Crying's for babies."

Letting yourself be convinced that you shouldn't feel as you do is like letting yourself be convinced that you shouldn't be so tall. If you were to believe that, what could you do? You could start off by feeling guilty about it and ashamed, and walk hunched over for the rest of your life, causing yourself immeasurable discomfort, pain and embarrassment. But you'd still be tall.

Emotions are natural, and denying them is unnatural. But letting your emotions rage out of control is unnatural, too. At a certain point you may have to take charge again. If you can't do it yourself, get a professional—a psychiatrist, psychologist, counselor or spiritual adviser—to help you.

Emotional problems are as real as physical ones, and they can make you just as sick if they are not treated. For deep, little-understood cultural reasons, many of us feel embarrassed about getting help for emotional dysfunctions, although we freely consult medical professionals concerning physical ailments. This attitude can exact a high toll in mental—and physical!—health. One common consequence of emotional extremes is fatigue, the central concern of this book. Here are some emotional problems most likely to cause or aggravate fatigue.

FRETTING AND FATIGUE

At any given moment, about 5 percent of all Americans are depressed. But if only those who suffer from chronic fatigue are included in the survey, the number soars to approximately 80 percent. It may be that half of those have fatigue caused by depression. The other half are depressed because of their fatigue, a common occurrence in patients with chronic fatigue immune dysfunction syndrome (CFIDS).

Some doctors lump most fatigue disorders under depression because they are so closely linked. But we know fatigue has other causes that must also be considered: stress, sleep disorders, nutrition, illness and CFIDS. Each has its own sources and responds to specific cures. All types of fatigue can be complicated by stress.

A number of illnesses or conditions, especially strokes, epilepsy and multiple sclerosis, also claim depression as a common side effect. So even though stress and depression are closely linked and may even share common biological and biochemical roots, they are separate problems.

A person under stress is like a rubber band stretched to the limit, taut enough to twang if you pluck it and likely to snap if you pluck it too hard. Think of a similar rubber band that has lost its flexibility, its ability to stretch. It is limp, formless, without strength and utterly useless for any function. That's like a person in deep depression.

What makes the distinction between stress and depression even more confusing is that many people suffer from both, with the two conditions stemming from the same emotional roots.

When people are under constant stress for a long period with no end in sight, they are at risk for becoming depressed over the very prospect of living the rest of their lives that way.

Before we get into depression-related fatigue, let's look at depression itself.

Everyone knows depression. We've all been there—and probably will be again. Usually it passes, maybe within a week or two of failing an important exam, or on the first sunny day after a gloomy spell, or many months following the loss of a loved one. Depression usurps the time necessary to run its normal course. But six months to get over a bad test result, a month to stop feeling lousy because of weather, a year of anguish due to a death is not a normal course. It's a sign of deep problems that should be addressed professionally.

Depression usually results from one or more of the Five Ds: dejection, despondency, discouragement, despair and dismay.

You feel an overall sadness, tinged with apathy and exhaustion. Any joy you once experienced is only a distant memory. Nothing has any value in your eyes. And the accompanying fatigue is not the sweaty exhaustion that follows exertion. You have the energy, but you just can't get motivated enough to use it.

In the midst of depression, you are apt to find yourself sitting on the couch and staring at a corner of the room, unable to get up, let alone take a walk. The irony of depression-based fatigue is that the fatigue would lessen if you could mobilize yourself to do something physically demanding.

Depression tends to develop in conjunction with life's major turning points or at times when life is most unsettled—during adolescence, during pregnancy and shortly after giving birth, at menopause, at the death of a loved one, at the loss of a job, after a major disappointment and at the end of a relationship.

Listed below are some additional factors that may help you to get a wider perspective on the ways major depression can affect everybody's life.

- Women are more susceptible to depression just before their monthly menstrual period begins. The Cleveland Clinic Foundation reported on a study in 1991 that showed that depression, chronic fatigue and premenstrual syndrome (PMS) often coexist in women seeking treatment for premenstrual distress.
- Relatives of depressed people are also more likely than others to become depressed themselves.
- A very small group—believed to be less than 2 percent of the population—consists of victims of a chronic disorder known as a depressive personality. These people are likely to get depressed over events that most others can ignore or forget easily. They are simply prone to depression, possibly

THE CASE OF THE DEPRESSED EXECUTIVE

Steve was an executive in a small but fairly successful business. He had a fulfilling life, a good income and a wonderful family. Though he could point to nothing wrong with his life, Steve was depressed. This was accompanied by a constant tiredness that fed off the depression. But since his life seemed to be going so well, he refused to accept the fact that he was depressed—at first.

Although the depression was constant, it intensified about every six weeks, to the point that Steve could not get up in the morning. Nothing mattered. Whether he went to work or not, got fired or not, all seemed irrelevant. He considered suicide.

The overwhelming combination of feelings, mostly sadness and apathy, just engulfed him. He cried and didn't know why. He hid so no one would see him crying. He couldn't sleep, and his attention span shortened. If he picked up a book, he lost interest after the first paragraph.

Steve's fatigue was a relatively minor problem compared with the sadness that seemed to swallow him whole. He knew his family couldn't understand what he was going through, so he shunned them. Communication seemed useless and futile and required more energy than he had. Anyway, what could he say?

After several months of living this way, Steve's depression seemed to lift slightly. He noticed that he had more interest in work and family, and he began to realize how serious his situation was.

With his wife's encouragement, Steve saw a doctor who diagnosed major depression and referred him to a psychiatrist. Through counseling Steve came to understand the nature and causes of his depression. A year later the depression was gone, along with the fatigue.

due to a chronic abnormality in the brain's neurotransmitters.

• Aside from the depressions that routinely hit adolescents, people between the ages of 25 and 44 are particularly apt to experience episodes of depression.

• Women are twice as likely as men to suffer from serious depression. Small wonder when you consider the events that can trigger depression and realize that men don't experience menstruation and pregnancy, postpartum stress or menopause.

• At least one in ten (some say one in five) Americans will suffer at least one case of major depression in his or her lifetime.

JUST A BAD MOOD, OR TRUE DEPRESSION?

The American Psychiatric Association says a person who shows at least four of the symptoms below nearly every day for at least two weeks is clinically depressed and should consider treatment.

1. Feelings of worthlessness, self-reproach or excessive or inappropriate guilt.
2. Indecisiveness or a diminished ability to think or concentrate.
3. Either poor appetite and significant weight loss or increased appetite and significant weight gain.
4. Either insomnia or significantly increased sleep.
5. Trouble thinking or moving smoothly or confidently.
6. Loss of interest or pleasure in usual activities, or decrease in sexual drive.
7. Fatigue and loss of energy.
8. Recurrent thoughts of death or suicide, or suicide attempts.

There are two basic types of depression. The first, exogenous or reactive depression, is a reaction to an event—the death of a loved one, loss of a job, separation or divorce, anything that causes you profound sadness. The second, endogenous depression, is caused by something inside you, and it's usually harder to deal with, generally longer lasting and more severe than reactive depression. Even worse, people who have this second kind of depression don't know why they're depressed; they just are.

As a result, people who go through endogenous depression can also develop terrible feelings of guilt or shame. After all, they see no good reason to be depressed. No one has died. They still have their family, their job, their belongings.

Ancient Greeks called endogenous depression *melancholia* and thought it resulted from an overabundance of a natural bodily fluid they named black bile. The more enlightened scholars of the Middle Ages knew that depression had nothing to do with black bile. The real cause of depression, they said, was demons from hell!

Demons of a more secular nature is one way to summarize Sigmund Freud's ideas about depression. He theorized that endogenous depression was the result of deeply buried, unresolved childhood traumas and conflicts—our childhood demons coming back to haunt us.

Today many doctors still think some depressions are caused by natural bodily fluids—not black bile, but an imbalance in the natural brain chemistry.

Like the rest of the body, the brain is mechanical, with nerves operating like the wires in a computer system. All bodily functions, from the movement of the hands to the beat of the heart, are regulated by nerves. So are thoughts and emotions.

The nerves are connected to each other by chemicals known as neurotransmitters. If these are unbalanced, the functions of the nerves are impaired.

One leading school of thought holds that depression is caused by an imbalance in the levels of neurotransmitters in the brain. This may be genetic (some families have a long history of depression), or it may be induced by external circumstances. It is possible that the foods we eat influence the levels of neurotransmitters in our brain and, as a result, our moods.

No one knows exactly what causes endogenous depression or why reactive depression lasts so much longer for some people than for others. But most experts do agree that depression is a result of combined biological and psychological factors that are not always possible to separate and unravel.

If you are depressed, whether or not you know why, you have to learn to deal with it. That might require outside help.

Depression can do more that just rob your life of joy, contentment, happiness, satisfaction and accomplishment. It can also kill you. Depression can end in suicide, the tenth leading cause of death in America.

While thousands actively commit suicide, many others just give up on life and let themselves die. Most of us can name people who died as a result of either active or passive suicide. Doctors treating people for depression are constantly on the lookout for suicidal tendencies in their patients.

Even though most cases of depression will eventually resolve themselves, there are ways to speed up the process: formal medical treatment, therapy and, in some cases, hospitalization (especially in cases where suicide is possible). All three forms of treatment can involve drugs, psychiatric counseling or a combination of both.

But even people with major depression can get some relief. Many therapists find that volunteer work, regular exercise and reprogramming negative thought patterns can go a long way toward pulling depressed persons out of their funk. These techniques and others are discussed in more detail in the following chapter.

TAMING UNFOUNDED FEARS

A study of 200 people with chronic fatigue done at the University of Connecticut School of Medicine showed that 26 of them, or 13 percent (ten times the national average), also suffered from panic disorder, simply described as a state of panic at an inappropriate time. For example, panicking at the thought of getting into an elevator when there is nothing wrong with the elevator, there is no one threatening inside of it, and there are no other signs of danger would qualify as a panic disorder.

In 21 of the 26 patients, panic disorder either preceded or developed with the chronic fatigue. Further study showed that a significant number of those with panic disorder had a history of severe depression as well as a lifelong tendency to have unexplained physical ills.

Some people are ruled by fear. And it doesn't make much difference if their fears are reasonable or not. These folks lead a limited and joyless life filled with stress and tension. They are trapped. The very thought of facing those fears and dealing with them can produce more panic.

Fear and panic are very stressful states. They drain your energy, prevent you from getting fully rested and nibble away at your energy reserves.

Some counselors who deal with fear look at it this way: F.E.A.R.—False Evidence Appearing Real. Instead of seeing what is really there or what is really likely to happen, people who are victimized by their own fears decide what the outcome will be and refuse to consider any other possibilities.

"If I go outside after dark, I will be mugged."

"If I don't do what the Smiths want me to do, they won't like me anymore."

MANIC DEPRESSION— EMOTIONAL PING-PONG

A manic-depressive careens between two emotional extremes: manic—energetic, gregarious, busy, ambitious and optimistic; and depressed—withdrawn, lazy, paranoid, hopeless and solitary. It's like going from the emotional north pole to the emotional south pole every so often, but on a predictable timetable for some.

In the manic state there is boundless energy and enthusiasm. A manic person stays up all night, cleaning the house or working on the car, and stands ready for the next day's activities. This can go on for weeks.

But this phase is followed by the polar opposite: severe depression, where all activity or desire to be active ceases.

This affective disorder, called bipolar disorder, is particularly difficult to treat because people want to cure only the unwelcome half of it. They'd like the manic or active state to continue. In some ways it is similar to cocaine addiction without the drug. The highs are a source of tremendous well-being, but they are always followed by corresponding lows that bring misery and self-doubt.

One key to overcoming a manic-depressive state is to recognize and accept the simple fact that happiness is meant to be a chronic condition. A true mountain climber, for example, enjoys the entire climb, not just the five minutes at the peak. So enjoy and appreciate the whole process of living, the ups *and* the downs, not just a few select moments along the way.

"If I tell people what I really feel or think, they'll never want to talk to me again."

"If I try anything new, anything at all, I'll fail."

Another way to spell *fear* is: *F*orget *E*verything *A*nd *R*un.

"I'll just move, find a new apartment. That will solve everything."

"If I change the subject and pretend I didn't hear the question, I won't have to answer it. And I'll say I have to leave because I'm late for an appointment."

Here are two tips for handling panic disorder.

1. Get hold of yourself. Tell yourself that the state of fear is worse than whatever it is that you are afraid of.

2. Face your fear with the support of a friend in a safe, controlled way.

For example, if you are afraid to ride an elevator, practice going near one with a friend you trust. When being near one no longer terrifies you, pick an off-hour and spend some time getting in and out without letting the door close. When you are comfortable with that, let the door close, but get off before the elevator moves to a different floor. Finally, ride the elevator up a floor and then back down. Then try riding it up more floors. Do this for a while, and eventually you'll be ready to ride an elevator whenever the need arises. Maybe it won't be in carefree comfort, but it won't be in terror, either.

Some psychologists work with different airlines to help people overcome their fear of flying. They take groups of phobic people onto an airplane and let them sit in it without taking off. While inside the aircraft, the psychologist heads a group discussion about fear of flying. After several of these sessions, most people in such a group, in which individual anxieties are discussed and unreasoned fears are often resolved, are willing to fly.

THE POISONOUS EFFECTS OF ANGER AND RESENTMENT

Anger and resentment go together like hay fever and sneezing.

You get angry at someone and either you get over it or it gets the best of you. That anger grows and festers and turns into an obsession. You can't concentrate on anything else. The anger spills over and affects everything you say and do. It can use up so much of your energy that there's little left for living your life.

We all know people who are perpetually angry—still mad about what Aunt Agatha said at Cousin Herman's high school graduation, or about the F they got in high school English, or at the spouse who died and left them to raise four young children on their own.

Anger is a normal human emotion. At times it is justified, but if anger becomes an obsession, you are in trouble. When you are angry with someone for a long time and spend your days resenting that person, you permit that person to live inside your head—rent free—trashing your most valuable property, peace of mind.

Among the many ways to get rid of obsessive anger, the simplest—but not the easiest—is to make a truce with the person. Visit or call Aunt Agatha and talk it over, or write her a letter. But do something about it.

It may be that, for you, the only way to get over anger is to wish the person well. Some people pray. And it does work. Pray in whatever way is comfortable for you. But do it—either pray for that person or in some way wish them well. It isn't necessary to have an emotional breakthrough with a deep change of heart; you just have to *do* it. You may not even be sincere when you start. But this kind of praying on a daily basis for two weeks will make your anger begin to go away.

Why should you do this for someone whom you'd like to see boiled in oil? For the simple reason that you need it as much as that person does. Your anger and resentment are preventing you from living a full, rich and energetic life. If you want your life—or your energy—back, you must get rid of your resentment or your anger. The only way to get better is to wish the other person well. (Those who are angry at someone who is dead—and many people are because they were left go on alone—should look at the section on grief later in the chapter.)

If you are angry at city hall or the IRS, or about the way your company operates or your boss runs the department, consider two simple questions: Is there anything you can do to make the situation better? If so, is the action reasonable?

Writing a letter to the person in charge is reasonable. Writing that letter on the side of their building with spray paint isn't.

Many people find a great deal of comfort as well as relief from anger and resentment in the Serenity Prayer (see page 132).

HOSTILITY IS SELF-INFLICTED RUDENESS

Hostility is anger in action, and it comes in two primary forms:

Overt hostility. Like a war, everyone involved knows there is a fight going on, and the weapons are in plain sight.

Covert hostility. Like diplomats, people may be smiling, but the daggers are present—hidden and sharp.

Hostile people know exactly what they are doing. Covert types pretend that their smiles are real and that any hurtful comment they make "just sort of slipped out, by accident. You know I'd never say anything like that on purpose. It was a joke, honest."

Some covertly hostile people don't realize what damage they are causing. In some cases the root of their hostility is buried so deep that they don't know why they do and say the things they do. They find no joy in it, and they often feel guilty, but they can't stop themselves. These people need help or counseling to discover the cause of their anger. Whatever the reason, and regardless of the type of hostility, the attacker is damaged as much as the target.

According to many doctors, hostility is hard on the heart and digestion. It can also interfere with sleep, rest and relaxation.

In summary, hostility acts like a combination of anger and stress to drain you of energy all the time.

WORKING THROUGH GRIEF

Grief is a perfectly natural reaction to loss, whether it be the death of a loved one, the loss of a job, a major disappointment or the breakup of a marriage, relationship or friendship. As we saw earlier, it can often lead to depression—and profound exhaustion.

The important thing to remember about grieving is that it takes time to run its course. It can take months, maybe even a year or longer. But our world moves too fast to allow for that. At work we're on the fast track; we eat fast food; we apply for instant credit, look for instant gratification, fall in love at first sight and so on. We tend to feel guilty about extended grieving: "Why is it taking so long?" The reason lies in the number of stages we must pass through in the grieving process: denial, anger, resentment and, finally, acceptance.

Therapists say you must go through each stage in turn. Trying to skip a stage, suppressing the feelings or pretending you're not affected just prolongs the sense of loss. Here is how it works with the death of someone you love, perhaps your best friend.

First you deny that she has died. You don't want her dead. You love her and need her. She is such a major part of your life that you can't imagine her not being there anymore. So you deny to yourself that she's dead.

Eventually you face the reality of her death. Then comes the anger. You have lost someone precious to you, and you are very, very angry about it. Maybe you scream at everyone you know, even blame them. Maybe you blame yourself. Perhaps you shout at God, blaming him for taking your best friend.

Soon your anger turns into resentment—directed against your dead loved one! How dare she die? How could she desert you, especially when you need her so much? A real friend would have stayed alive. She wouldn't have abandoned you.

At last you achieve acceptance. Your friend is dead. You still feel the loss from time to time, but you are ready to go on with your life. You can even look at her photo and remember the happy times together without going to pieces.

So let yourself grieve. Talk to others about your feelings. Ask how they got through their grief. The pain is there, and if you don't let yourself feel it and work through it, you'll never get free. It will drag you down and steal your energy. In this case, fatigue is a direct result of trying to hide from your emotions.

Take an honest look at yourself and recognize all the emotions present in your grief. This lets you begin to resolve your feelings. Once you do that, the energy you need to hold them at bay will be released.

EMOTIONAL EARTHQUAKES EAT UP YOUR ENERGY

Strong emotions can produce instant stress. The stress levels that come with several years of living with a teenager who wants to be a drummer in a rock-and-roll band—or any teenager, for that matter—can be equaled or even surpassed by one major argument with your spouse, a close call in traffic, a registered letter from the Internal Revenue Service or a 3:00 A.M. visit to the emergency room. All of these can get the adrenaline pumping and the emotions jumping. And they all demand a great deal of energy.

When the event is finally over, you are drained. The greater the emotional high, the longer the hangover; the longer the hangover, the deeper the energy drain.

While you can stop speeding and thereby avoid getting tickets, it's unlikely that you have as much control over your emotional responses to life. The main thing to remember is that periods of high emotion are followed by periods of low energy.

The occasional emotional hangover is as normal as the occasional sleepless night, upset stomach or head cold. After all, no one is 100 percent healthy 100 percent of the time, and that goes for emotional as well as physical health.

The best you can do is to prepare for these emotional earthquakes and learn how to spot the early tremors. On occasion you might even decide these outbursts are worth it to air pent-up feelings or to settle an issue that will only get worse unless it is resolved.

If ever you are suffering from an emotional aftershock, be nice to yourself. Take it easy. Don't expect too much from yourself that day. After all, you are recovering from a jolt to the system that is as real as a physical one. You will get through it.

You can also learn a lot from the experience—from the upheaval itself, the emotions that trigger it and anything else that comes to light as a result. Stirring up the emotions is like stirring a big pot of stew. You never know exactly what will rise to the surface.

CHAPTER 13

Blues Busters

It's clear from the preceding chapter that serious depression often requires professional help that might include antidepressant drugs or counseling. But what about mild or moderate depression, the sort that keeps you (and up to 25 percent of your fellow Americans) down and out for a few days or a week every month? What do you do when you feel the blues coming on?

In chapter 11, we looked at a number of simple, practical and effective ways to deal with stress. Some of them might be useful for dealing with depression, too. If you can handle that, you automatically reduce the amount of fatigue you feel.

Developing a more positive outlook on life might help you get rid of mild or moderate depression completely. And if you are truly seriously depressed, the following tips could bring some relief. Just remember, none of these ideas will work unless you want them to. You must make up your mind that you want things to change, or they won't. If, consciously or unconsciously, you prefer staying depressed and pitying yourself, that's exactly what you'll do. But if you want to get rid of the blues and start living again, you can—if you know how.

In case you wonder whether depression actually is the source of *your* problem, consider these three common signals. Depressed people:

- Tend to isolate themselves. They want to be alone, so they cut themselves off from the world. They are likely to skip work and miss appointments. If you insist on being by yourself, you are in bad company.
- Focus on their own condition, ignoring the world around them.
- Have trouble recognizing the truth about their situation. Either they exaggerate its severity and complain to anyone who will listen or, martyrlike, they remain silent about their pain.

If you see yourself in those quick clues, here are some ways you can work against the grip depression has on you.

- Get out of the house. Get to work on time. Go out to lunch. Go shopping. Take a walk.
- Pay attention to what's going on around you. The longer you focus on yourself and your own depression, the longer you will remain depressed. Transfer your concerns to something else for a change.
- Tell the truth. Let people know what's going on inside of you and how you actually feel—good or bad, happy or frustrated—and listen, expressing your interest and concern, when others tell about how they feel.

Getting out, paying attention and telling the truth are good tools for busting up the blues. But if those aren't enough, here are some other ideas that work for many people.

DO A REALITY CHECK

Take some time to do a quick inventory of your world. Is anything actually wrong?

Ask yourself questions like these: Are you sick? Are you broke? Is a loved one seriously ill? Are you grieving because someone you care about has died? Has someone hurt your feelings? Did you wrong a friend? Are you menstruating, or due to begin? Are you going through menopause? Are you losing your hair? Have you put on weight? Are you going through a divorce? Do you get enough sleep? Have you lost your job? Did someone important to you forget your birthday? Are you feeling old?

We all have some unpleasant elements in our lives. Could it be that such a situation is the source of your depression? ("I don't know" is a valid answer to that question.)

You don't have to know why you're depressed. Even if you don't know the true cause, you can at least rule out some improbables. And by the process of elimination, you can begin to define general areas where your problem might lie. Every bit of knowledge is helpful.

If and when you actually do figure out why you are depressed, the next question is: "Can I do something about it?" If the answer is yes and the action is reasonable, take it.

Even if you can't actually resolve the problem, just identifying it can help you determine how serious it really is. You can also reject the consequences of the problem.

GO AHEAD—PITY YOURSELF

If you're depressed, let yourself wallow in it soulfully and sorrowfully—for 15 minutes. Set a kitchen timer or an alarm clock to let you know when the torture time is up.

Take those 15 minutes to feel all the misery, pain and anger you have inside of you. If you feel like crying, cry. If you feel like yelling, yell. If you feel like swearing, swear.

Feel sorry for yourself; bask in it. Tell yourself just how unfair the world is. Put a sad song on the compact disc player. If you want to sing the blues, go ahead.

As soon as the alarm rings, your time is up. If you still feel sad or blue, try one of the other blues busters. Then get on with the rest of your life.

LIST YOUR EMOTIONAL ASSETS

When you're depressed, it's hard to think about anything in a positive way. "Sure," you say, "every cloud has a silver lining, but the silver's all tarnished in my cloud, and I'm the one who has to polish it."

You've done your reality check. Now make a gratitude list. List at least ten things you are thankful for. Start off with the fact that you are alive. If you can't think of anything else to add, answer these questions.

- Is there a roof over your head?
- Do you have food in the refrigerator?
- Are there clothes in your closet?
- Is your house warm and comfortable?
- Have you paid the rent or mortgage?
- Does someone love you?
- Do you have good friends?
- Have you a favorite song? Movie? Color? Food?

Your gratitude list accomplishes three primary objectives:

- You see, in black and white, just a few of the blessings in your life.
- It helps you focus on the positive instead of the negative.
- It helps motivate you to make a serious effort to get rid of the blues.

A gratitude list doesn't get rid of problems, nor does it minimize any of the real trials you face; it just gives you a break from them.

We all have problems—physical, financial, emotional and spiritual. We have problems with the people we love, those we work with and others we see every day.

Problems are part of life. Sure, they get us down, but we don't have to stay down. Use your gratitude list to give yourself a lift.

ELIMINATE "SHOULD" AND "SHOULD NOT" FROM YOUR VOCABULARY

Early in his career, comedian Woody Allen quipped, "Life is what happens while you're making other plans."

As a rule, when you make plans you use the words *should* and *should not* a lot ("By age 35 I should be heading my division at work" or "My children should not have trouble in school if I work with them"). After all, your plan has to conform to your desires, your standards and your likes and dislikes.

So when real life happens—when some of the "shoulds" don't happen and the "should nots" do—you can get depressed quickly. Hey, this is not the life you planned!

If you spend more time accepting reality and living life on its own terms instead of trying to get it to conform to yours, your days are easier, more fun and a lot less depressing.

This also applies to your relationships with other people. Don't hold others to your impossible expectations.

Take *should* and *should not* out of your vocabulary and see how much things improve in your contacts with those around you.

BANISH THE "BUTS"

So you've made your list and are reminded that your kids love you. Then you slip right back into depression, saying, "Yeah, but . . . they haven't called me in weeks."

Or you see that your refrigerator is full, and then it's: "What if . . . I don't have enough money to buy food when I retire in 20 years?"

"Yeah, buts" and "what ifs" get you nowhere but back into depression.

Stay in the present. Accept that you can't change yesterday, and tomorrow hasn't arrived yet.

Stick to today's gratitude list, without any qualifiers.

TREAT YOURSELF WELL

List three things that you can do today—either immediately or a little later—that would make you happier than you are now, make you laugh or give you a feeling of satisfaction.

You might, for example, take a walk, call a friend, play a game, watch children playing, have a nice meal, rent a video, pursue a hobby, read a book, plan a vacation or a weekend away and so on. Do at least one of these today, and be ready to do another one tomorrow.

The key here is to write down things that you can—and will—actually do, not something you know is impossible. So do not list things like losing 25 pounds in 25 days, writing a hit play or getting a hole in one, for that will only lead to frustration.

DARE TO CHANGE

Maybe you feel tired because you're in a rut or bored with your life. If one day is pretty much like the next, the lack of stimulation can leave you spent and dull.

Try something new—an exotic recipe, a fruit or vegetable you've never had before. Buy a new scarf or tie. Rent a foreign movie. Make new acquaintances. Start a new hobby. Take a class. Learn a language. Make yourself an "expert" on something, anything.

It's hard to get out of a rut because boring, miserable and depressing as it might be, at least it's comfortably so. There's no threat to living in a rut because there's no change.

Change requires risk, and risk involves the possibility of failure. But look at it this way: If the worst happens you'll feel depressed, but since you're already depressed, what do you have to lose?

OPEN UP TO THE ENERGY AND EMOTIONS OF OTHERS

As a rule, depressed people don't communicate well with those around them. In fact, this failure may be an underlying cause of their depression. Even if it isn't, lack of communication can aggravate the problem. It can leave a person feeling alone and isolated. The isolation can lead to depression—and that is a major cause of fatigue. Anything that contributes to isolation or depression can add to fatigue.

Try expressing your feelings honestly. If you're uncomfortable about how to open up, start with something simple—an honest, positive statement to someone you love or trust. Do not expect any reward (though you will probably find one). Do it just because you want to and because it's true. It can be as simple as "I like the way you're wearing your hair today" or "I like that necktie. Is it new?"

Do not retreat from human contact. Be honest in your relationships, and use your ability to communicate your feelings in order to help those relationships grow.

Be willing to communicate physically. We need social, emotional and physical contact with other people. We need affection. Make it a goal to get—and give—at least three hugs every day.

Nurture honest communication like a delicate flower. In time you will feel comfortable about sharing your feelings. You will eventually develop the ability to share negative feelings, even with people who intimidate you now.

IF YOU DRINK, CUT DOWN OR STOP ENTIRELY

Alcohol is a depressant. It makes the central nervous system slow and less efficient. The initial buzz or feeling of euphoria that can accompany a drink comes with shutting off inhibitions and anxieties. The more alcohol, the greater the shutdown.

Alcohol interferes with coordination and clear thinking. Eventually it interferes with your ability to think at all. Regular consumption of more than a drink or two can also leave you deficient in the B vitamin thiamine or replace other, nutrient-rich foods and beverages, undermining your physical health. If you customarily head for the fridge and reach for a cold beer after a long day at the office or a hard workout, consider drinking a juice sparkler instead. You'll get an extra dollop of potassium, known to play a role in muscle endurance, and a little useful carbohydrate to perk up your brain. Tonic water with a twist of lime (but no gin) is another refreshing alternative. You may find that after sipping your nonalcoholic "relaxer," your urge for a bottle of beer—or several—will have passed, and you can plan a more productive, less energy-sapping afternoon or evening ahead.

People who drink to "cheer up" because they're depressed are fine as long as they stop after one or two—a glass of wine, a bottle of beer or a gin and tonic, for instance. But if they continue, they only compound their mental depression and leave themselves open to physical problems—memory impairment, an accident, liver damage and so forth.

People who drink when they are already taking tranquilizers, antihistamines or sedatives risk their lives: The additive effect of one drug (alcohol) on top of another can literally shut down your brain. Common sense says that if you load your system with alcohol and drugs that depress the central nervous system, you're not going to have the energy you need to be productive, creative or truly happy.

Studies show that half of all traffic fatalities, one-third of all traffic injuries, one-third of all mental health disorders and one-third of all suicides are alcohol related.

COULD THE PROBLEM BE IN YOUR MEDICINE CABINET?

It's quite possible that more people are hooked on "legal" drugs than on illegal ones—legal drugs like sedatives, muscle relaxants, cold remedies, painkillers and thousands of others. Many people don't realize that prescription and over-the-counter drugs can cause or aggravate depression.

If you take any medication at all, consult the *Physician's Desk Reference,* found in most libraries, to find out what the primary effects and side effects are. If the side effects are not listed on the container, talk to your pharmacist or ask for the patient-information insert. If you take several different drugs, check with your pharmacist to see how they interact.

If the medications you use are a problem for you, discuss it with your doctor. Perhaps he or she can switch you to another drug, decrease the dosage or suggest a nondrug alternative.

FAKE IT TILL YOU MAKE IT

Act as though you aren't depressed.

This doesn't mean you stifle your feelings. Share them with a close friend or counselor, or write about them in a journal. You can even feel the pain. Then move beyond it. Accept your depression and ask yourself, "What would a person who isn't depressed do in this situation?" And then *you* do it!

If you fake it long enough—put on the proverbial happy face—pretty soon you will actually feel happier. The depression may still be there, but it won't ruin your day. You'll be able to deal with your negative feelings on your terms.

It's just as Abraham Lincoln once said: "Most folks are as happy as they make up their minds to be."

EXERCISE FOR ENDORPHINS

As mentioned in chapter 11, exercise is a great way to reduce stress. It is also a great way to relieve depression and anxiety.

Exercise causes the brain to produce endorphins, chemical compounds that occur naturally in the brain and bring on a natural high. The more you exercise, the more endorphins you produce. That's how people get to experience a "runner's high" during a long run.

Studies show that a brisk walk of 15 or 20 minutes, or any form of aerobic exercise, can bring more short-term relief from depression or anxiety than a session with a psychiatrist—and it's cheaper. Not only that, but the more depressed or anxious you are, the better you'll feel after a workout, especially an aerobic one.

If you're not up to anything too strenuous at first, start off by just walking outdoors in nice weather. When it's too hot, too cold, too windy or too wet, find an attractive, enclosed shopping mall to walk through.

Nine holes of golf is also good exercise—unless you spend it riding around in a golf cart. Walking the course is part of the fun and the exercise. Or design a home program with some exercise equipment like a stair-climbing machine or exercise bicycle.

If it's something more strenuous you want, try biking, hiking, jogging, running, in-line skating (if you have the knees for it), square dance, cross-country skiing, downhill skiing, volleyball or tennis.

As an added benefit, going for a walk or run or working out takes your mind away from your anxiety or the emotionally crippling self-obsession of depression.

You have many ways to exercise informally during the day. If you have a choice between the elevator and stairs, take the stairs. If you can walk to work, do so. If you have to drive, park farther from work than you usually do. The walk will do your body some good and clear your head as well.

Regardless of the type of depression or anxiety you have, any kind of exercise helps, whether it be low-impact aerobics, weight training, a session on a stair-climbing machine or just a pleasant walk.

It's not a total cure, of course, but the good effect of exercise is reliable. You will actually feel more energetic, refreshed and optimistic afterward.

Physical activity relieves the day-to-day blahs as well as long-term depression or anxiety, and it works for people of all ages. As an added bonus, exercise is good for your entire body. And it's unlikely that you have to worry about mild exercise conflicting with a medical treatment program. Still, it's best to check with your doctor.

DO A GOOD DEED

Helping others is a great way to help yourself out of depression. Studies conducted at Bowling Green State University and at New York State Psychiatric Institute, among others, show that extending a hand benefits the helper as well.

For reasons scientists don't yet understand, doing a kindness for another triggers the same endorphins set off by exercise. This results in the same sort of "high" runners enjoy.

Volunteer work provides more than a momentary rush of pleasure. According to a survey of volunteers in Canada, those who participated on a regular basis over several years actually felt healthier and less stressed than a similar group of nonvolunteers.

What you do (it should be something you enjoy) is as important as the amount of time you devote to it. And it doesn't have to take all your free time for you to benefit. Studies show that 18 percent of Americans do at least four hours a week as volunteers. But two hours a week appears sufficient to trigger the endorphins and reduce stress, depression and fatigue.

If you can't take on scheduled volunteer work, get imaginative—do a good deed for a friend, neighbor or relative. Even something as simple as a cheerful phone call to someone who is housebound will be a plus for both of you.

MORE SUPPORT CAN BOOST YOUR ENERGY

Alcoholics Anonymous, Al-Anon and other 12-step programs are based on the "kinship of common suffering." People who have or who have had similar problems get together and share not only their experience but, more important, their strength and hope.

If you are being treated for depression, ask your doctor or counselor if it would benefit you to talk to another patient. If so, ask the caregiver to help arrange it. Also, many social service agencies have listings for various mutual-support groups and can tell you how to contact the group that serves your needs. They might even help you start your own.

If you join with fellow sufferers, you can get and give more than emotional support. You can also learn some practical tips for coping with and getting through your depression.

LAUGH AT LIFE

Laughter, like exercise and volunteer work, causes the release of endorphins, those wonderful brain chemicals that pump up energy levels by producing a natural high. As the long-running feature in *Reader's Digest* says, "Laughter is the best medicine." Doctors, psychiatrists, psychologists and other medical—and spiritual—professionals agree.

As we saw in chapter 11, it's good for stress. It's even better for fighting depression.

When you laugh, you affirm that you are not alone, that you are alive and part of the human race. It proves that you are also able to recognize and admit just how silly you and your fellow human beings can be.

Besides, it is impossible to concentrate on two things at once, so a person who is busy laughing is too busy to be depressed.

But what will make you laugh? That's for you to say. We all have a sense of humor, but sometimes we misplace it, even intentionally. We resist the fun of laughing because it will get us out of our sour mood, and we are secretly enjoying the self-pity and martyrdom. Or we feel that we are too important, too serious and too cultured to laugh. Baloney!

If you haven't laughed in so long that you've forgotten what will tickle you, turn on the TV and see if the sitcoms do it for you. If not, try cartoons, and look for the characters from the golden age of animation: Bugs Bunny, Road Runner, Daffy Duck and that crowd.

If you can't find anything funny on TV, go to a video store and check out something with the Marx Brothers, Charlie Chaplin or Laurel and Hardy—any of the old classics. Pick out some stand-up comedy videos or "Saturday Night Live" collections. Try several different comics, both old and new. And when you find a comic or comedy troupe you like, get more of their work.

Go to a library or a bookstore and browse through the humor section. Page through cartoon books or the works of Dave Barry or

Roy Blount, Jr., until you find a few that get you laughing. Take them home.

Spend an evening at a comedy club; check the yellow pages if you don't know where to find one.

One caveat: If you're suffering from depression, humor that relies on cynicism or the hardship of others may do more harm than good. Under those circumstances, good-natured humor may be more salubrious than dark humor.

Your sense of humor is like a muscle. If you don't use it, you lose it. And in the same way that physical exercise will help you get rid of unwanted fat, laughing will help you get rid of depression.

Depression is an emotion as natural as joy, anger and love. It becomes a problem when it dominates your life and drains you of the energy you need to live your life to the fullest.

If you suffer from both chronic fatigue and depression, eliminating the depression will ease your fatigue. It will also give you the determination needed to deal with the other issues that contribute to your fatigue.

CHAPTER 14

How Nutrition Figures in Fatigue

Your body knows what and how much you should eat, and it tries to tell you this by the way it gains and loses weight, by your complexion, by your overall mood *and* by the energy you have. Specific foods and compounds can have a direct effect on your fatigue level.

A key point in any discussion about nutrition and fatigue is that your body constantly changes and so do you. You can be physically, mentally and emotionally affected by whatever happens to you or to the people you know and care about.

There are no hard and fast rules—"Take this pill and eat these foods and be healthy and happy forever!"—but there are some basic guidelines you can use that have proven effective for most people over the centuries.

Even though they hate to admit it, relatively few doctors really know much about nutrition as it relates to health, much less its effect on fatigue.

Typically, a practicing physician assumes that a patient's nutrition is "normal" if the patient shows no weight problem nor any obvious diet-related ailment such as rickets, anemia, scurvy or beriberi.

The notion that a person could be made even healthier, have more energy and get more out of life by taking diet supplements of iron, vitamin C or magnesium might not occur to the average physician. Unless a person is sick, why would he or she need supplements?

As a group, physicians spend little time investigating the potential nutrition holds for renewing energy, even though it's axiomatic that food is essential to energy production.

In the same way that some doctors have to be forced to think of fatigue as a serious medical condition, many have to be forced to consider that certain changes in diet or nutrition can help overcome fatigue.

Medical science rightfully demands strict criteria for health claims. Without such controls, medicine would risk its credibility. But it's clear that health information is not yet complete in all areas. This is especially true of chronic fatigue. In particular, we know relatively little about the effects of nutrition on chronic fatigue, and there are no obvious answers. While I haven't personally done any strict medical studies on this theory, I am convinced that attention to diet is essential in treating chronic fatigue.

Granted, there is no consistent dietary pattern in patients with chronic fatigue immune dysfunction syndrome (CFIDS). Nor are there any predictable changes when the illness is treated with specific diets. Healthy athletes who consciously follow a good diet are as likely to come down with CFIDS as couch-potato junk-food addicts. What's more, CFIDS is only one type of chronic fatigue. Even if improved nutrition does nothing for the disease itself, improving nutrition—like reducing stress—may somehow ease the symptoms of the illness.

Nevertheless, as we saw earlier, poor nutrition can definitely cause some types of chronic fatigue. And certain things will invariably worsen chronic fatigue: alcohol, too much sugar and, in some cases, excessive consumption of dairy products.

When it comes to fatigue, the term "poor nutrition" has a very broad meaning. It includes eating too much of one thing and not enough of another, or eating either at the wrong time. So let's start by looking at some examples.

LOSE POUNDS, LIGHTEN UP

Because of the consequences it can bring, obesity is the number one health problem in America today. Experts estimate that 20 to 40 percent of the public is overweight. Most doctors define obesity as being 20 percent heavier than the recognized norm among others of the same height and body type.

Everyone is aware of the risks that come with being overweight: heart disease, diabetes, circulatory problems and bone and joint disease, for example.

Ironically, many overweight people lack the nutrients it takes to produce all the energy their bodies require. In other words, overweight people get more than enough food; the problem is, they eat too much of the wrong foods.

The relationship between excess avoirdupois and chronic fatigue is simple: The more weight you carry, the more energy you require to carry it. Even when you are lying down, breathing takes more energy because there is more chest tissue for your diaphragm to move.

In my practice I've seen plenty of people improve their energy level and their self-esteem by losing weight. One CFIDS patient I was treating who lost 30 pounds showed a marked improvement in overall energy levels. Although the CFIDS was not cured, it became easier to live with.

When it takes a large part of your energy to breathe, digest, walk or even sit up, there isn't much left for anything else. Overweight people also get winded by the least bit of exertion—climbing a flight of stairs, running to catch a bus, pushing a cart through a crowded supermarket or unloading groceries from the car.

Generally the fatigue associated with extra poundage is the gentle, nagging type of tiredness that people grow accustomed to, and they get used to the slow-moving life that comes with it. But many also notice a new fatigue, such as the type that accompanies diabetes mellitus, hypothyroidism, CFIDS or any other condition. The problem is, physicians who treat overweight people for fatigue tend to treat the weight problem alone, without looking for other possible causes.

The bottom line: If you're too heavy, losing weight is a key component of a fatigue-free program.

And you can start by adding fat reduction to your diet goals. The North American diet averages 30 to 45 percent fat. Cutting that to 20 to 25 percent is a major step toward losing weight, as is generally reducing the amount of food you eat.

The next step is to burn more calories. Your weight level results from the rate at which your body burns the calories you consume—your metabolic rate, which is different for everyone. That's the reason people with a slow metabolism get so frustrated when they fail to lose weight on a strict diet, while others with a faster metabolism eat so much more without gaining an ounce.

Even though the metabolic rate is basically genetic, people with slow rates are not necessarily doomed to obesity. The good news is that diet combined with exercise will do the job, too.

Even if obesity is not the main reason for a person's fatigue, losing excess weight will alleviate the tiredness and even make it easier to find the other causes.

DON'T STARVE YOURSELF OF ENERGY

Being slim is one thing; being emaciated is quite another. Eating less than 1,000 to 1,200 calories a day will leave you malnourished due to lack of protein, calories and essential fat. And you'll have no pep whatsoever.

But even normal dieting can cause some fatigue.

How much body fat is healthy *and* attractive? Take an honest look at yourself. Then check the weight range for someone your age, sex and height. (See the table on the opposite page.) If you don't even make the lower range, you just might be anorexic. Such folks have very little energy, but due to the psychological aspects of anorexia, they deny it. They will tell you they have the energy, but they just can't be bothered. They're lying.

CHECK OUT NUTRIENTS YOU NEED, STARTING WITH PROTEIN

Some people are so used to feeling poorly that they don't realize there's an alternative. In fact, it is only after they start feeling really good that they recognize how badly they felt before.

Are You Overweight?

New government guidelines give a more realistic range of desirable weights for adults. Use this table to help determine how close you are to "ideal weight"—one that is conducive to good health *and* high energy levels. (Women should refer to the lower end of each range given; men should use the upper limits as a guide.)

HEIGHT	WEIGHT IN POUNDS*	
	19 to 34 Years	35 Years and Older
5′0″	97–128	108–138
5′1″	101–132	111–143
5′2″	104–137	115–148
5′3″	107–141	119–152
5′4″	111–146	122–157
5′5″	114–150	126–162
5′6″	118–155	130–167
5′7″	121–160	134–172
5′8″	125–164	138–178
5′9″	129–169	142–183
5′10″	132–174	146–188
5′11″	136–179	151–194
6′0″	140–184	155–199
6′1″	144–189	159–205
6′2″	148–195	164–210
6′3″	152–200	168–216
6′4″	156–205	173–222
6′5″	160–211	177–228
6′6″	164–216	182–234

*Without shoes or clothing

THE CASE OF THE TIRED VEGETARIAN

Sarah was 27 when she first noticed increasing fatigue over a six-month period. To climb a full flight of stairs, she had to stop and rest twice. She was confused and bewildered by her fatigue and changed her lifestyle to improve her health.

Sarah had always been troubled by cramps and excessive blood loss during her menstrual periods, so she was used to it and paid it little attention. She had become a vegetarian about a year earlier to reduce her cholesterol level.

A number of people had told her that vegetarian diets were very healthy, provided that she include milk products, rice, beans and peas in order to get the necessary protein. She followed her new diet faithfully: She ate neither eggs nor meats. And she avoided leafy green vegetables because she didn't like them.

Because of her progressive fatigue, Sarah saw a doctor who gave her a complete physical. Routine blood tests revealed that she was suffering from iron-deficiency anemia. She wasn't producing enough blood cells because she didn't have enough iron in her diet. Her condition was complicated by the excessive loss of blood during her periods.

Sarah began to take iron supplements, and she added iron-rich foods to her diet. Her energy and vitality quickly returned. And yes, she is still a vegetarian.

This tendency toward accommodation makes it hard to decide on the body's true needs concerning essential nutrients.

Furthermore, different people have different metabolic needs. For some a diet heavy on snacks and fast foods provides all the vitamin B_{12} they can use. Others require much more B_{12} to fight off pernicious anemia.

What it all comes down to is this: Despite the many advances, studies and breakthroughs, the precise amount of any one compound an individual person needs for optimum health is still a matter of guesswork.

Remember, this is a book about fatigue. So, even though we're looking at the broad range of vitamins, minerals and other nutrients, the focus is on fatigue.

Proteins are made up of amino acids, the body's major building blocks, involved in the structure and function of all the major organs. We know the body produces some of its own amino acids (called nonessential), but others (essential) must be part of the diet.

Researchers are learning that the amino acid balance is extremely important to the body's energy production cycle. Any upset can lead to fatigue.

How much protein should the average person consume in a day? Estimates vary, but it's safe to say at least 45 grams. That must include the *essential* amino acids, those the body cannot make. The best way to ensure getting enough essential amino acids is to eat a balanced diet that includes protein-rich foods such as veal, lean beef, poultry, milk and dairy products, nuts, grains, peas, lentils and beans. All proteins are not the same, so eat a variety of them. If you give your body a good mix, it will balance them out properly.

Don't assume that meat should be your primary source of protein. In fact, it shouldn't. Beans, lentils and grains make good sources because they're fat free. For example, a cup of soybeans contains more protein than three ounces of beef, veal or chicken. Millions of people around the world consume a healthy and balanced diet that is entirely meat free.

STARCHY CARBOHYDRATES DRIVE THE HUMAN MACHINE

Carbohydrates (starch and sugar) are our primary food source, and eating them is the easiest and most economical way to get energy. That's because all carbohydrates are converted to glucose, the sugar the body uses to produce energy. Some is burned for immediate energy needs, and the balance is converted into fat to be used for energy later. While some authorities state that carbohydrates do not convert into fat easily, others say that carbos can end up on the waist, thighs or buttocks.

Most Americans get about half of their total calories from carbohydrates. But current research shows that the distribution should be 60 percent from carbohydrates, 20 percent from protein and 20 percent from fat.

Starch (consisting of hundreds of glucose units, which the body makes available for energy) is found in potatoes and other vegetables as well as grain products such as spaghetti, bread and crackers. Sugar (fructose) occurs primarily in honey and fruits.

As an added attraction for those who must fight fatigue, starchy carbohydrates offer relief from the tiring effects of stress. Researchers at Muguley Hospital in Fort Worth, Texas, note that starchy carbohydrates help the body produce serotonin, a brain chemical that exerts a calming, relaxing effect in stressful times.

THE SUGAR BLUES

The problem that comes with heavy sugar intake is that our perception of what a normal energy level actually is—or should be—is altered. It's like blowing up a balloon, then letting the air out. There's plenty of action as it zigzags around the room. But that's over fast. Then the empty balloon just lies there.

That's akin to what happens when you eat sugar-laden foods. But the crash that follows a sugar rush doesn't necessarily mean you're having a serious sugar low (a threat to those with diabetes), also known as hypoglycemia. It only means that your body has returned to normal after flying so high that "normal" seems low. People who do not have diabetes but who do have hypoglycemia usually tremble and get weak, tired and hungry.

In day-to-day living, sugar-based fatigue is relatively mild and intermittent. After a sweetened breakfast accompanied by coffee or tea—with sugar—there is a burst of energy. You might feel as though you could jog five miles, no sweat. But later in the day, once that sugar high vanishes, you feel a nagging listlessness, perhaps best described as a loss of enthusiasm.

In other words, it all evens out. Sugar brings you up, and it also takes you down. The more you ingest, and the more often you do so, the farther you fall afterward—and the longer you stay there.

Certain people are hooked on sugar. Without it, they get tired, cranky and nervous. They crave that jolt.

Sugar fatigue is no mystery. Many people depend upon a sugar high to get them through those stresses at work and at home. They accept the reality that a crash is inevitable. But they are sharp when they need to be sharp, so it is worth the exhaustion that follows.

There is a deeper and possibly more dangerous aspect to the sugar high. With time, the quick energy effect is muted. Eventually you need ever greater amounts of sugar to get the same effect, and the more you take, the more damage you do to your entire system. It's like burning high-octane gasoline in a car that wasn't built to take it. It will burn the engine out. Your body requires a steady supply of nutrients for smooth performance; it wasn't designed for a diet heavy in high-octane sugar. By burning too much sugar, many of these nutrients, such as the important B vitamins, are depleted and lost. Your entire body suffers.

TRASH THE FAT

Dietary fats produce a lot of energy when they burn and a lot of trouble when they build up in our bodies. That's because our bodies metabolize fat differently than they do carbohydrates.

Fats are not converted to blood sugar but are broken down into their essential components, called fatty acids, and enter the energy chain. Those not needed for immediate body energy are turned into body fat at once. So unless you spend considerable time on fat-burning activities—such as running, walking or working out—the fat tends to build up like a reserve.

There are two basic classes of fats: saturated fats, most of which come from animals and are usually solid at room temperature, and unsaturated fats, which usually come from vegetables, nuts and fruits and are liquid at room temperature.

Most experts believe excessive intake of saturated fats is a major cause of heart disease and obesity among Americans. On average, we consume 37 to 40 percent of our calories from fat. Reducing that to 30 percent or less could help lengthen your life and lower your weight.

Although you may need to reduce your fat intake, you cannot do without fat. It is an essential part of your diet. Without fats (and the fatty acids they break down into), the body won't work properly. But you need only a tablespoon or so a day—45 to 55 grams, at the most.

VITAMINS MAKE THINGS HAPPEN

The word *vitamin* was coined in 1914 by Casimir Funk, a Polish-American biochemist who was studying the compound we now know as thiamine. He first called it *vita-amine*—an organic base, *amine,* that was vital to life, *vita.*

Scientists have known for nearly 200 years that the body requires more for life than an adequate supply of amino acids, proteins, carbohydrates and fats. But Funk was among the first to figure out exactly what those elements were and where to get them.

While the body can synthesize much of what it needs, it cannot make its own vitamins. (It cannot produce some necessary trace minerals, either. We'll look at those a little later.)

Vitamins come from the food we eat—with one exception. Vitamin D is sometimes called the sunshine vitamin because it is produced in the skin during exposure to the sun. A few foods, like mackerel, also contain some vitamin D.

Very little is known about treating CFIDS with vitamins. A number of researchers do use very high doses of vitamin B_{12} and vitamin C, according to *Treatment News,* a publication of the CFIDS Association. While there are still no careful studies that prove this to be effective, I have seen patients improve and regain lost energy while taking these vitamins. This measure calls for careful consultation with a CFIDS specialist.

Otherwise we can only extrapolate from what we know: Fatigue is a common sign of vitamin deficiency.

Vitamin A (retinol). Because of its importance to a healthy retina and clear vision, vitamin A is also known as retinol. It occurs either as the vitamin itself or as beta-carotene, a food substance that the body converts into vitamin A.

The best sources of vitamin A are carrots and other orange and yellow fruits and vegetables like cantaloupes, sweet potatoes and winter squash as well as dark-green leafy vegetables such as kale and broccoli.

Treatment News also reports that studies show fish oil will improve energy levels in patients with CFIDS. No one really knows why, but many think it may be due to the abundant vitamin A that fish oils contain.

Vitamin A is necessary for vision, cell growth and cell differentiation, and it helps to prevent night blindness. There are indications that it might also reduce the risk of heart disease and strokes, plus breast, cervical, colon, lung and prostate cancer. Vitamin A might also retard the development of macular degeneration, a common cause of blindness among the elderly.

Thiamine (vitamin B_1). You'll find this vitamin in peas, beans, wheat germ, yeast and meats. But prolonged cooking destroys thiamine. That's why so many foods are fortified with it.

A lack of thiamine can lead to beriberi, a disease characterized by fatigue, weight loss, numbness in the extremities, unsteady walking, memory difficulties and heart failure. Chronic alcoholics are often thiamine deficient.

Riboflavin (vitamin B_2). Milk, egg whites, liver and leafy vegetables are major sources of riboflavin. Since liver is quite high in cholesterol, you're better off relying on greens (or skim milk) for this nutrient.

The lack of riboflavin can result in skin disorders or lesions—inflammation of the tongue and cracked skin around the corners of the mouth, a characteristic of many CFIDS patients. And we know that a riboflavin deficiency will also cause exhaustion.

Vitamin B_6. The prime sources for B_6 are meats, poultry, fish, fruits, nuts, seeds and vegetables. Vitamin B_6 helps prevent anemia, skin lesions and nerve damage. A deficiency of B_6 can also cause fatigue, disorders or lesions, inflammation of the tongue and cracked skin around the corners of the mouth.

Vitamin B_{12}. To beef up your B_{12} supply, flesh out your diet with lean meats, nonfat milk products and fish. Vitamin B_{12} is best known for helping to prevent pernicious anemia, a condition that is commonly identified with fatigue.

Many believe that large doses of this vitamin may improve energy production even if you don't have a deficiency, and some doctors treat fatigue by injecting high doses of B_{12} into the muscles. This amounts to using it as a drug, not as a vitamin. If you're exhausted and want to consider this option, look for a knowledgeable physician who can realistically assess the potential of such a treatment for you. It doesn't work for everyone, but approximately 30 percent of CFIDS sufferers treated this way report improved energy levels.

Biotin. This water-soluble vitamin, found in many meats and nuts, is necessary for certain enzyme reactions in the body. Taking large amounts of antibiotics and, more rarely, eating raw eggs will deplete biotin, and a shortage can cause fatigue, depression and a scaly skin eruption. So if your doctor has put you on antibiotics for any reason, ask about the need for shoring up your biotin supply.

Vitamin C (ascorbic acid). Most people automatically think of citrus fruit when they think of vitamin C, but it occurs in many other foods, primarily green peppers, strawberries, raw cabbage and green leafy produce. Vitamin C fights infection, hemorrhages, gum disease and scurvy, a rare disease (once common among sailors deprived of fresh foods while at sea) characterized by fatigue, muscle weakness and tenderness, and bleeding. Stress depletes vitamin C levels, and so do smoking and exposure to cold.

Although vitamin C was not actually identified until 1930, its effects have been known for hundreds of years. North American Indians are credited with teaching early settlers what foods to eat in order to prevent scurvy.

Some physicians and nutritionists recommend daily vitamin C tablets to help prevent the common cold—or to get it over with quickly, although the effectiveness of this has never been shown conclusively. Many also believe that vitamin C will help the body cope with stress and disease, which can cause or aggravate fatigue.

This vitamin is also used as a treatment for fatigue, but with mixed results. Some patients report increased energy, while others report no change at all.

Unlike some other vitamins, vitamin C cannot be stored well in the body for later use. So it's essential to consume plenty of foods rich in vitamin C every day.

Niacin (nicotinic acid). Plentifully contained in grains, meats, fish, nuts and various beans, niacin prevents a skin disease called pellagra, an ailment characterized by fatigue and weakness.

Although full-blown pellagra is rare in North America, mild forms of it do occur occasionally, and even the mild cases cause fatigue.

Vitamin E (alpha-tocopherol). This fat-soluble vitamin occurs in meat, poultry, nuts, seeds, whole grains, leafy vegetables and fish-liver oils. It helps prevent anemia.

Folate. This plentiful nutrient is especially abundant in mushrooms, yeast and green leafy vegetables. It is vital to the body's chemical operations, including energy production. Alcohol and certain antibiotics tend to interfere with its activity. So if you drink alcohol regularly or take antibiotics, you should consider using a folate supplement.

MINERALS MAKE A MAJOR DIFFERENCE IN ENERGY

As we all learned in high school chemistry, the minerals and chemicals contained in the human body could be bought from any chemical-supply house for less than $10. But if you lack any one of these essentials, it could mean thousands of dollars in medical costs as well as pain, suffering and fatigue. Of course, it's important to get the proper amount. An overdose of certain minerals can be as damaging as too little and can result in serious health problems.

Iron. If you eat such foods as liver, beef, lamb, chicken, raisins, vegetables, grains, beans, nuts, fruits and eggs, you're sure to get enough iron for normal needs. Iron plays a major role in our ability to build and maintain energy levels. It's the element that lets red blood cells carry oxygen to the tissues for use in the energy production cycle.

Despite the wide availability of iron, some people fall short. Many have given up liver and eggs—for good reason. Others skimp on other iron-rich foods for various reasons. A shortage leads to iron-deficiency anemia, one of the most common diseases in the world. It's also a major cause of fatigue. But eating iron-rich foods is only part of the solution. What you eat with them is also important.

Vitamin C helps the body absorb iron. So drinking orange or tomato juice or consuming other vitamin C-rich foods, such as peppers, with iron sources, such as beans and rice, makes a lot of sense. For additional iron intake, you can do what your grandmother did: Cook with cast-iron pots and pans, which pass on small amounts of iron in the food they hold.

On the other hand, drinking coffee or tea with an iron-rich meal interferes with the body's ability to absorb the iron. Milk and other high-calcium foods have the same negative effect.

Iodine. Found in iodized salt and seafood, iodine is essential to the health of the thyroid gland. A lack can lead to hypothyroidism, which is likely to cause severe fatigue.

Magnesium. Vital for every cell of the body, magnesium is an essential ingredient in the energy cycle. Although it is plentiful in beans, nuts, vegetables and meats, deficiencies are common; when severe, they can cause confusion, convulsions and muscle rigidity. Recent findings show that the red blood cells of patients with CFIDS are low in magnesium.

In 1991 the British medical journal *Lancet* reported a study in which a group of CFIDS patients with low levels of magnesium in their red blood cells were treated with injections of magnesium. More than half had improved energy levels. But other researchers following up on these experiments questioned whether the level of improvement was in fact due to magnesium treatments.

Many CFIDS researchers can point to specific patients who had a gratifying response to magnesium. So while it doesn't seem to help everyone, it does work for some.

FOOD ALLERGIES, A PRIME SUSPECT IN FATIGUE

Many people have a violent reaction to specific foods, food additives or even food colorings. They break out in hives or have trouble breathing, for example. Others are merely "sensitive" to certain foods, and their reactions are more subtle—perhaps mild fatigue or loss of energy.

An individual might be allergic to just about anything, but the most common food allergens include shellfish, fish, corn, nuts, peanuts, legumes, eggs, chocolate, cow's milk, citrus fruits, wheat, tomatoes and MSG (monosodium glutamate).

Milk and other dairy products. Most of us know of someone who is slightly allergic to milk, and two predictable symptoms of that allergy are depression and fatigue. Other people are strongly allergic and their reactions are more severe.

As we get older, our bodies tend to lose some of the digestive enzymes that break down milk solids in our intestines. This leads to digestive problems such as accumulated gas, constipation or diarrhea.

Even young children can have problems digesting milk. Some have slight intestinal bleeding, resulting in loss of the iron the blood contains. If this happens often, the child can become anemic.

On the plus side, milk is a good source of protein, calcium and phosphate, and a valuable food for those who tolerate it well.

But as mentioned, the calcium in milk can interfere with your body's ability to absorb iron. So if you do drink milk—or if you take a calcium supplement—avoid doing so at the same time you take an iron supplement or eat iron-rich foods. Otherwise they will bind together and cancel each other out.

If you think dairy products are a factor in your fatigue, eliminate them for a week or so. Then try them again, watching for familiar and uncomfortable signs of an allergy, such as diarrhea and stomach pain. If you develop either symptom, you might want to skip dairy products for a while and test them again periodically.

You can also substitute soy milk or soy-based cheeses for dairy products and see if the problems stop. Lactose-free milk is also available. Of course, that's convenient if you have lactose intolerance, but it won't necessarily solve an allergy problem.

If you don't like the taste of lactose-free foods, or you want to avoid the expense or the bother of looking for them, you can buy enzyme tablets (such as Lactaid) that will help you digest the lactose in regular milk and dairy products and avoid unpleasant reactions.

Wheat, rye and oats. Eating large amounts of wheat, rye and oats—in breads and other baked goods or breakfast cereals—can also cause fatigue because these foods all contain gluten, a common allergen. Some people become tired or anemic or develop a condition known as celiac disease (which damages the intestinal tract) due to gluten.

The most common symptoms of gluten intolerance or sensitivity are a loss of appetite, weight loss, fatigue, anemia and bulky, light-colored and fatty stools. The degree of the symptoms depends upon the degree of sensitivity.

If you suspect you have a problem with gluten, go without foods that contain it. Gluten-free foods are available from health-food stores. You can also write to food manufacturers for a more complete list of gluten-free products.

It's important to remember that all vitamins and minerals contribute to health and energy. Their lack can lead to specific disorders, and fatigue is very often one of the symptoms.

Do you get enough vitamins and minerals? It all depends on what day it is and whether you have a cold or are feeling run-down, how busy you are and what's in the refrigerator, how much junk food or sugar you've been eating, and what demands are being placed on your mind and your body.

What should you do? Most of us have learned over the years that the minor inconvenience of buckling up our seat belts can save our lives in an accident; so can looking both ways before crossing the street. In the same vein, taking a daily all-in-one vitamin/mineral supplement could be another important safety measure as well as a cheap form of health insurance.

Try it for a month and see if it makes a difference in your life. Maybe it will, maybe it won't, or maybe you'll decide that you need even more. It's your choice, but consult with your doctor before taking megadoses.

In my own practice, I emphasize sound nutritional practices for all my patients, especially those with chronic fatigue. While I have not been using megadoses of vitamins or other nutritional supplements, I do know that other researchers do. In fact, some treat CFIDS exclusively with nutritional therapies. While many claim good responses, there are still no medical studies that prove the effectiveness of many of those strategies.

But there are definite nutritional steps you can take to help fight your fatigue. We'll consider them in the next chapter.

CHAPTER 15

The Fatigue Fighter's Diet

Some people are always watching their weight and dieting to be slim, but they don't eat enough of the right kinds of food, nor do they eat when they should for consistent strength. The foods you prepare, how you prepare them and when you eat them—all are vital elements in defining your energy levels.

We also know that some people are terminally tired all the time, certainly too tired to cook a meal. But this doesn't mean that they are doomed to takeout, TV dinners, fatty, high-calorie snack foods, frozen pizza or cold cereals at every meal. We'll tell you what you need for good eating and how to make sure you get it.

First we'll quickly review the food elements that help fight (or induce) fatigue. Then we'll look at some high-energy meals rich in desirable elements that are also quick, easy to prepare and suitable for company, too.

CARBOHYDRATES, THE ENERGY CORE

For long-term energy, stoke up on carbohydrates—both simple and complex—which the body converts into energy.

Sugar is a simple carbohydrate, the kind that's found naturally in a glass of orange juice as well as the refined stuff you might add to your morning coffee.

Starch, a complex carbohydrate, is the type found in cereals, potatoes and rice.

Most nutritionists recommend that at least 50 to 60 percent of your calories come from carbohydrates, primarily the complex kind. Many athletes on rigorous training schedules up their carbohydrate consumption to as much as 70 percent of their caloric intake.

The body needs both, but timing counts when it comes to consuming carbohydrates.

Sugar (simple carbohydrates). As mentioned in chapter 14, sugar provides quick energy. But like a fireplace filled with crumpled newspapers, it burns hot and fast and then it's gone. You get a burst of energy, but no more. In an hour or less, you're tired again.

Sometimes a quick jolt is all you need to finish a long tennis match, pedal the final few miles of a bike race or get through a complex morning meeting, and a glass of pineapple juice, a candy bar, a piece of chocolate or any other concentrated sweet will give it to you.

The efficiency with which your body turns sugar into energy has both a plus and a minus. The plus is that a shot of sugar (a candy bar or soda) really does rush into the bloodstream and in minutes gives the brain a wake-up call that gets you through an energy crisis beautifully. (Of course, the more sugar-based food you ordinarily consume, the more you need to get a real kick.) But on the minus side, you can't depend on sugar to fight fatigue for very long—for a full afternoon of concentrated work, for example. The body simply won't permit that.

In a healthy person, that rise in energy-giving blood sugar is reduced to normal by the action of the hormone insulin. The body releases precise amounts of insulin in order to level off any fast blood-sugar rise as soon as possible. When that happens, the energy zap that got you over the hump vanishes even faster. In some people, feelings of fatigue and changes of mood follow in the wake of sugar consumption. You may feel sleepy and tired (not necessarily weak) a short while after a sugar snack.

For someone plagued with a chronic lack of energy, this is not a desirable state.

Starch (complex carbohydrates). Starch also offers an energy burst, but it takes hold more slowly and lasts longer than sugar. That's because the body doesn't absorb starches as fast as it does sugar.

Have an English muffin with jelly and you get double-duty results: a fast shot of energy from the sugar in the jelly or jam, plus a longer-lasting boost from the starch in the muffin.

PROTEIN FOR THE LONG HAUL

The body absorbs protein more slowly than it does any form of carbohydrates. Protein also lasts longer, once absorbed.

If we take our English muffin and jam and add a slice of lean meat, or have it with a glass of skim milk, the protein in the meat or milk will kick in after both the sugar and starch have done their part. In this regard, protein is a basic building block of a fatigue-fighting diet. A lingering cold, chronic fatigue or general weakness are just a few signs that suggest a possible protein shortage, according to Liz Applegate, Ph.D., lecturer on sports nutrition. Protein foods give you the right stuff to fight off disease and to build, repair and maintain all types of tissue. See our 30-Day High-Energy Program at the end of the book for tips on how to ensure that you're getting enough protein to meet your everyday needs and ward off nutritionally related fatigue.

HOW FAT SAPS YOUR ENERGY

One reason we like fat so much is that it takes a long time to digest. That additional period makes us feel full or satisfied longer. But that full and heavy feeling can also drain our energy, so that we think more about napping than about any activity requiring real power.

While fats are an important part of your diet, no more than 10 to 20 percent of your calories should come from that source. Be particularly careful to avoid saturated fats found in butter, whole milk and full-fat cheese, ice cream, beef fat (in steaks and burgers), hydrogenated vegetable oil (used to prepare baked goods and fries) and coconut and palm oil (in some crackers and snacks or other prepared foods). They have been cited as high-risk factors in heart disease and stroke.

FOOD SUPPLEMENTS AND GOOD SENSE

Vitamins and minerals are an important part of the process that converts food into energy. What's more, individual nutrients contribute to a fatigue-fighting diet in very specific ways, as explained in chapter 14. Both vitamin and mineral deficiencies can result in chronic fatigue, says Dr. Applegate, particularly shortages of the B vitamin thiamine and the mineral iron.

A note about supplements: A single multivitamin/mineral tablet (or a supplement program) might do a lot to improve your energy levels. It is important to remember, however, that men and women have some gender-related nutritional needs (pregnancy and menstruation, for example). What's more, nutritional requirements also change with age.

Overdosing on certain vitamins (particularly fat-soluble ones such as vitamins A, D and E) and certain minerals is also linked to fatigue. So before you go overboard with supplements, check with your doctor about what's right for your age, sex and medical history.

POWER-PACKED MEALS WITH MINIMAL EFFORT

Knowing which foods will help you gain or maintain your energy is important. If you can afford to eat most of your meals out or have them brought in, or can enlist someone's help to cook (and clean up afterward), more power—and energy—to you.

But what if you're the one who does the grocery shopping, then plans and prepares the meals? How do you get it right—plenty of nutrients, not too many calories or too much fat, yet tasty, easy and fast?

To help you out, here are some ideas, tips and techniques for quick and simple meals that fill the bill.

Cook in gallons, serve in pints. When you have the time and the inclination, cook a lot. It's usually as easy to make two or three gallons of stew, soup, sloppy joes, chili or spaghetti sauce as it is to make enough for one meal. The same can be said for meat loaf, casseroles, taco filling, lasagna, even hamburger patties (all with lean meat and minimal added fat, of course).

Once you've made the sauce or the dish, divide it into single-meal portions and put them into freezer containers, the sort you

HELP FROM HIGH-ENERGY SNACKS

A number of high-energy snack bars are available to help sports enthusiasts sustain their energy while hiking, bicycling or pursuing other activities. Can these snack bars help you out with an endurance feat of your own—a sales meeting late Friday afternoon, perhaps?

They could be worth a try. Look for a bar that gets more than 70 percent of its calories from carbohydrates and less than 10 percent from fat. The rest should come from proteins. In her book, *Power Foods,* Liz Applegate, Ph.D., lists three bars that meet those criteria: Exceed Sports Bar, NuTreat and PowerBar. Check the label on other bars for high fat and high calorie content, two negatives if you're watching your weight or cholesterol. Choose the bars highest in vitamins and minerals.

Don't rely on energy bars on a daily basis, though. The emphasis should be on maintaining a steady supply of all-around nutritional energy sources all the time. Concentrate on fruits and starch-based snacks such as muffins and crackers as long-haul, antifatigue measures.

can take right out of the freezer and pop into the microwave or defrost quickly and heat on the stove.

You can even make several pounds of individual meatballs, freeze them on a tray, then place the frozen meatballs in freezer bags. Later, you can pull out as many as you want for a meal.

Spaghetti or pizza, it's the same wonderful sauce. Some sauces work well for very different dishes. Spaghetti sauce, for example, doubles as pizza sauce. Infused with your own creativity and special ways of preparing ingredients, the sauce might turn up in an aromatic chicken cacciatore, a honey-and-garlic-flavored meat loaf, a lusty eggplant casserole or a wide variety of other meals.

Snack cool, crisp and light. Melons and other sweet fruits and vegetables are also sources of quick energy. They are loaded with natural sugars that can provide a midmorning or midafternoon energy boost.

If you're extra tired—or extra busy—buy precut fruits and vegetables for salads, stews and stir-fries at the salad bar or produce section of your local supermarket. Think of the grocer's salad bar as a take-out restaurant. Put a scoop or two of fruit salad on top of nonfat or low-fat yogurt or cottage cheese for a high-energy lunch, quick and effortless. If you want to enhance the appeal of a cold plate of fruits or vegetables, serve them with a dip of low-fat yogurt or nonfat sour cream, or spice up cool cucumbers and crunchy raw cauliflower florets with a zingy salsa dip.

Prepare a delicious cold salad by heaping cooked pasta—spirals, shells, elbows—in a bowl and tossing in some drained kidney beans, peas or Italian green beans. Top it off with a jar of pimentos and a jar of artichoke hearts in olive oil.

Rice really is nice. Start with a bed of precooked rice, then add a bag of precut mixed Chinese vegetables and sliced broccoli from your supermarket salad bar. Spread the vegetables over the rice, then zap it all in the microwave for a quick, vitamin- and carbohydrate-rich energy-boosting meal.

To be sure you always have some precooked rice on hand when you need it, order an extra carton or two the next time you have Chinese takeout.

Pita pocket power. Another way to use Chinese vegetables is to stuff them inside a pita pocket, then heat the sandwich in your microwave. Or use Italian vegetables and cheese instead. Pita pockets keep well in the freezer, so you can stock up.

Do-it-yourself frozen pizzas. If you are less than fond of storebought frozen pizzas, make your own. Just start with the frozen pizza shell, or use toasted bagels or English muffins as the base for individual pizzas. Add diced pineapple, lean chicken or diced ham, asparagus, cauliflower or broccoli and various types of peppers or mushrooms (pizza sauce is optional). Bake your creation until crispy.

This kind of food is a great source of long-lasting carbohydrate-generated energy, a first-rate weapon for fighting fatigue.

Iron in meats and sweets. Dark-meat chicken is an iron-rich food, but the body may not absorb all the iron available from it. To improve iron absorption, stir-fry diced chicken with red peppers or broccoli, or pan-grill fajita-style tomatoes, green peppers and onions, lightly seasoned with cumin or coriander. The vitamin C in the vegetables will help your body absorb the iron.

Satisfy your sweet tooth with a handful of raisins or dried apricots, especially if you're worried about anemia. Both are iron-rich snacks, and you need iron to keep up energy.

Energy-rich Mexican mix. For another quick and healthy Mexican meal, prepare some quick-cooking brown rice. Then use your microwave to heat chili con carne. Serve the chili over the rice. It takes just a couple of minutes to prepare, but the complex carbohydrates in this combination will keep your blood sugar level up for hours.

Fish in a flash. Fish cooks quickly, and it's a snap to prepare. Wrap single-portion servings of thick fish such as haddock, cod, catfish or even shark in aluminum foil, adding parsley or other compatible herbs, a slice of lemon or lime and maybe a sliver of onion. Seal the foil and either bake or grill about 10 to 15 minutes, then serve immediately.

No-fuss baking. Buying is the fastest route to no-strain baking. Look for an in-store bakery, but opt for fresh-baked whole-grain bread or muffins instead of those tempting sugary goodies. If that won't do it, go for uniced angel food cake, gingersnaps or molasses cookies (all are generally lower in fat and cholesterol).

However, preparing a fresh, homemade dessert doesn't have to be an all-day chore—and the finished product doesn't have to be fattening. Here's the simplest of the simple: Core some Stayman (or any tart) apples, and stuff them with a mix of raisins, brown sugar and a pinch of cinnamon. Bake until soft and serve.

CHAPTER

16

Exercise: The Surprising Prescription That Really Works

It sounds like a joke. Exercise—the single most valuable treatment for *fatigue?* But that's exactly what it is, according to certain researchers.

In almost every authoritative publication devoted to chronic fatigue, exercise is listed as the treatment most likely to work as a healer.

Your body—the very one you've been dragging around for so long—is your best ally in getting a move on. Depending on the underlying cause of your fatigue, the mechanism for shifting from "park" into "high gear" may be hard to resist—once *you* turn on the ignition.

Robert S. Thayer, Ph.D., describes this phenomenon clearly in his book, *The Biophysiology of Mood and Arousal.* He envisions a young man sitting quietly under a tree on a summer's day. He will soon push a lawnmower, but at the moment his body's processes are in an energy-conserving pattern of quiet.

Now he gets up to mow. At once his whole body is transformed from a state of peaceful rest to one of readiness for vigorous action. Just the decision to get started busies the brain as it plans the job; the nervous system advances from a state of rest and recuperation to one that mobilizes the body for action. Hormones are released to increase metabolic rate and speed heart action.

Then the young man pushes the mower. Now his heart pumps faster, circulating more oxygen and energy-carrying glycogen. Blood pressure rises, and breathing gets deeper and faster to bring in more oxygen and expel more carbon dioxide. The young man's bodily motor is purring.

Many other positive internal changes also kick in, but our main interest lies in what happens to this individual's vitality quotient. As the youth continues mowing, Dr. Thayer says, he gradually develops "feelings of energy, vigor and peppiness." It just happens! The sheer act of exertion seen in our healthy example sets in motion changes that overcome fatigue.

There are a few exceptions, however. In some situations—which we'll discuss shortly—exercise actually aggravates exhaustion.

CAN EXERCISE HELP BOOST YOUR VITALITY?

At this point you're probably wondering whether the exhaustion that's been plaguing *you* is exercise-friendly. Will a few jumping jacks or a short jog build you up, or will exercise knock you out?

Generally speaking, exercise is a plus whenever chronic tiredness is rooted in stress, depression, a sleep disorder, some type of medical condition or a nutritional problem, particularly one related to obesity. But when the exhaustion can be traced to chronic fatigue immune dysfunction syndrome (CFIDS), exercise is usually the wrong way to go. In fact, the negative effect exercise has on CFIDS is so common that doctors tend to equate the presence of this hard-to-identify disease with the worsening of symptoms brought on by exercise. (Exercise can also play a positive role in treating CFIDS, and that will be discussed later in this chapter.)

So in order to determine if and how exercise fits into your own personal fight against fatigue, you need to know why you are so tired in the first place. Here are some common causes of fatigue and some suggested strategies for using exercise to fight them.

Step up your activity, peel off pounds. If being overweight is a possible source of your fatigue, exercise is a surefire treatment. Virtually every specialist in the field agrees that exercise is a necessary part of any effective weight-loss plan. It helps to burn calories. And as the excess pounds slide away, the energy once needed to tote those pounds around becomes available for other endeavors. As a result, fatigue becomes a faint memory.

Aside from that, activity improves the body's ability to convert the food you eat into energy—another phenomenon in your favor. Your muscle tone toughens up with training, so you get greater results from less work.

No question, action is the ideal antifatigue strategy when obesity is at the bottom of the problem.

The perfect tonic for stress. Any long-term tension can be a major drain on your energy supply. But you can use workouts to plug that leak. Here is how the cycle works.

In stressful situations, the body pours out profuse amounts of catecholamines, the hormones that trigger the fight-or-flight reaction. But as vital as these hormones are in the right situation, the stressed personality demands the nonstop emission of these crisis chemicals in *all* situations. That means the body is kept on edge and wired for action indefinitely. No wonder stress brings on energy burnout—there's no breather, no time to regroup.

Exercise, on the other hand, provides a clearly defined reason for producing catecholamines: You need the energy it takes to swim five laps in the pool or do 20 push-ups. That's the "on" switch. This is followed by rest and a slowdown that puts out that fizzy hormone mix as energy returns to tired muscles. That's the "off" switch.

Unless the flow of those chemicals is capped, your body doesn't get a chance to build up a new supply of energy, so you are trapped in a prolonged state of fatigue. Working out helps to reset the fatigue/rest equation by tiring muscles to the point of normal weariness, then resting them properly so more new energy can accumulate. You can see why exercise is an essential in a true stress-reduction program.

An added benefit of antistress exercise is its potent role in putting out cigarettes—for good. Since stress tends to trigger the urge to smoke for so many people ("I'm so upset, I've got to have a cigarette!"), what licks stress is bound to work against the smoking habit, too.

I always recommend walking as an antianxiety exercise. It's better than aerobics, running or lifting, in my opinion. For one thing, it uses all the muscle groups. But more than that, it lasts longer; you have time to unwind, get a change of scene, be distracted from immediate concerns. And you can do it anytime, at any pace.

No exercise is *wrong* for cutting into stress. But walking has it all, and no experience or training is necessary.

The mood elevator that works. You might call depression and chronic fatigue the terrible two of the emotional world. Like high winds and heavy rains, they combine to make big trouble for anyone in the way. However, just by bringing exercise into the picture, you gain the strength to get out of their path.

The trick you must master—and it's not a simple one—is to overcome the lassitude and indifference that stifle the will to work out. Even a small start will result in a proud sense of well-being and generate still more activity. For openers, take a walk. People who suffer from depression report that this pleasant effort makes them feel hopeful and energetic.

A convincing demonstration of the way exercise can work its magic on depression comes from a study conducted by Robert Brown, Ph.D., and others at the University of Virginia, reported in *The Physician and Sports Medicine.* Six hundred volunteer students were included, about 120 of whom were clinically depressed. The entire group, observed over ten weeks, was divided into six sections: depressed students who did no exercise, those who exercised three times a week and those who exercised five times a week, plus three similar groups of students who were not depressed.

Whether normal or depressed, students who chose not to exercise showed no decrease in depression at the end of ten weeks. But in the four active groups, both normal and depressed students who jogged a minimum of 30 minutes showed a highly significant reduction in depression scores (the five-times-a-week joggers registered a "quite impressive" reduction). All exercising groups also showed significant reductions in hostility, anxiety, stress and fatigue. Equally impressive, all exercisers registered increases in cheerfulness and *energy.*

These findings were no surprise to Dr. Brown, who has been testing the moods of students since the 1970s—nearly 5,000 men and women participated. This huge sampling has consistently shown that exercise is related to decreased hostility, anxiety *and fatigue* as well as improved energy and sleep.

Some kind of exercise is an indispensable part of the treatment for depression and the fatigue that comes with it. And the good effect builds upon itself. The more you get out and move about, the more you want to get out and move about.

I once had a patient who came to me convinced that his fatigue was due to CFIDS. But because of the pattern and type of fatigue and the lack of other CFIDS symptoms, I suspected that depression was the real problem. When he became uncomfortable as I asked him questions about his personal life, I was even more confident that my observation was correct.

I suggested a trial of exercise as a "diagnostic" test. If he had CFIDS (or if he had both depression and CFIDS), the exercise would aggravate the fatigue and flulike achiness, possibly in a dramatic fashion. But this man got a tremendous lift from following the exercise program. Over the next several months it became obvious that the more he worked out, the better he felt. He did not have CFIDS, and after two or three months he was able to begin focusing on the obstacles that were making his personal life difficult.

A new way to control diabetes. The medical books list fatigue as a known symptom of diabetes, right up there with the other classic markers like excessive thirst and frequent urination. Most physicians agree that exercise is helpful in treating the disease, particularly among patients who are overweight. Because of the possible complications caused by overweight, weight loss—through diet and exercise—is important for such people.

If you have diabetes, don't start any vigorous exercise before checking with your doctor. For one thing, circulatory problems or heart disease can complicate diabetes, so any exercise program for people with such conditions must be individually designed.

Remember, your body uses more sugar when you exercise, so your blood sugar level tends to drop and should be monitored. Professional athletes who have diabetes are vitally aware of the need to accommodate their sugar requirements to the sport.

Many people with diabetes need special counseling plus adjustments in medication to prevent complications due to vigorous exercise. (Your doctor can easily say if this is a requirement for you.) As exercise lessens the severity of your diabetes, your lack of energy should diminish, too.

Exercise now, sleep later—and better. Show me a person who is tired all the time and the first question I ask is "Do you get enough sleep?" The answer I've learned to expect is "No."

EXERCISE TO IMPROVE YOUR PROFILE ON THE JOB

You're sure you could do a really good job at work, if you just had the energy to pull it off! Well, regular exercise can resolve that problem for you. Just enroll in a fitness program at a health club, attend the employees' gym at work or even style your own workout plans at home, and you're on the way to fatigue-free shifts and a real chance to move up the ladder.

According to a report released in May 1992 by the Association of Quality Clubs, a group that represents 2,000 health clubs, workers who exercise:

- Produce more. Four out of five workers at Union Pacific Railroad credit exercise for increasing their productivity and improving their concentration on the job.
- Are more decisive. Researchers at Purdue University who studied 80 people over a nine-month period found that the ability to make complex decisions improved 70 percent among those who began to exercise during that time.
- Show up for work. Absenteeism was cut by nearly half (45 percent) among General Electric employees who exercised, compared with those who didn't. Exercise among workers at other organizations (Du Pont, the Dallas Police Department and General Mills) also improved work attendance anywhere from 14 to 80 percent.
- Stick with the company. Fitness participants are 13 percent less likely to change jobs than others, Tennaco reported. Over a seven-year period, Canadian Life found that those who exercised were 32 percent less inclined to jump ship.

T. Boone Pickens, chairman of Mesa Petroleum, believes that "fitness is an essential part of the best-run companies." By extension, that means fit employees are the most prized workers in an organization because they have the energy to do the job better than almost everybody else. That energetic employee could be you.

Why don't these people get the rest they need? Well, some are overweight, which frequently leads to those two sleep bandits, snoring and apnea, the interrupted supply of oxygen to the lungs. (See chapter 9.) Others are stressed and resort to sleep-inducing medications, which can actually worsen sleep disorders.

Do you recognize these culprits? They're present largely because sufficient exercise is absent!

Light exercise in the early evening helps with insomnia, producing a mild, relaxing kind of tiredness that helps you drift off to sleep at bedtime. It's the perfect preparation for sleep. Medical studies show that regular, moderate exercise on a daily basis improves the quality of sleep in general, with fewer awakenings during the night.

THE SPECIAL ROLE OF EXERCISE IN TREATING CFIDS

As suggested by the earlier example, the relationship between CFIDS and exercise is unique. Any physical activity at all must be carefully tailored to the individual patient. While just the right amount of exercise is helpful, too much makes the symptoms worse. Not all medical authorities agree on this point, however. In fact, some even prescribe exercise (inappropriately, in my opinion) in the medical articles they write. Here we will show you an easy way to determine the amount of exercise that's right for you if you have CFIDS.

Caution is the watchword. It's important that a person with CFIDS remember to approach exercise warily. Even a light session of step-ups, arm rotations or just walking might trigger a relapse (worsening of symptoms) the next day. That setback might persist for several days before you can regain the preexercise level you achieved. (Researchers have yet to determine exactly why this worsening-by-exercise phenomenon occurs, but those familiar with CFIDS agree that it does exist.)

If you suspect that you suffer from CFIDS, beware if your doctor prescribes exercise as part of your treatment. Some well-meaning but uninformed physicians routinely recommend exercise to combat unrelenting tiredness, even when they know CFIDS is the basic cause. The consequences may be devastating to the patient. Carefully supervised, individualized activity, planned by a physician very familiar with CFIDS, is the only way exercise can work to aid a CFIDS patient.

Don't become a zombie. Now here comes a seeming contradiction: It is a mistake for a person with CFIDS to avoid exercise completely. As the symptoms of that ailment begin to subside, the tolerance for exercise rises ever so slightly. But that's a far cry from having the resources for an all-out effort! After months of inactivity, it is a mistake to hurry into heavy exercise. Caution and patience are called for here. Your body will tell you how strenuously you can exercise when dealing with CFIDS.

If you want a more definite directive, use this rule of thumb: Exercise gently to the point where the aching and flulike symptoms that characterize CFIDS flare up—then stop. Do not try to push through these feelings as you might if you were fighting depression. This very kind of "going beyond" the warning symptoms might bring on a relapse and open the door to even worse symptoms.

Recognize safe limits. The amount you can safely perform may also vary from day to day. Pay attention to the signals your body sends. And don't assume anything about the state of your progress.

For example, you might be able to walk briskly for 10 minutes one day and 20 the next. But you can't assume that you're ready for 30 minutes the third day. Progress very cautiously. At the first hint of muscle ache, lymph gland soreness (often at the groin, underarms or side of the neck) or that all-too-familiar feeling of impending exhaustion, stop and rest.

I had the opportunity to treat several professional athletes who were suffering from CFIDS. When such highly motivated and well-conditioned individuals develop the disease, it is obvious that the symptomatic fatigue they complain of is not due to stress or depression. They become very frustrated at the inability of their team physicians to diagnose the reason for their fatigue. Yet they learn quickly from experience that they can't continue to do any serious exercise. It may take a year or two of inactivity before they begin to feel real improvement as their illness subsides. On two occasions, I have seen athletes try to get back in shape too fast, and both times the athletes suffered a severe relapse as a consequence.

Feel your way. Your limits may vary from day to day. So whatever you do, don't try to "push the envelope." But don't let yourself be totally intimidated by the idea of exercise because you have CFIDS, either. Actually, it's better to attempt some activity and have a mild flare-up of symptoms than to live in fear of a relapse and spend your life on the couch. For most people with CFIDS, exercise does not make the illness itself any worse, only the symptoms. So if a workout aggravates your fatigue and discomfort for a few days, just do a little less the next time. Eventually the CFIDS is likely to subside to the point where a mild workout can be tolerated. Then you must feel your way as you gradually increase your efforts to a level where the first signs of pain or exhaustion show, then stop.

In truth, the ability to exercise defines the cure in CFIDS. As a CFIDS patient improves, that person reaches a point where real exercise can be tolerated without a return of symptoms. To me this signals a complete cure.

Unfortunately, many CFIDS patients resolve their symptoms and actually feel relatively well, but then, for some reason, exercise provokes a new flare-up. For them, exercise that tests their limits is appropriate, but if it aggravates their fatigue, they are still classified as recovering victims of CFIDS.

Concentrate on consistency. The key to any exercise program is steadiness. It is better to walk 15 minutes a day on a regular basis than to sprint half a mile once a week. In the 30-Day High-Energy Program at the end of the book, we provide an exercise program that is appropriate for most people with fatigue, whether it is due to CFIDS, stress, depression or medical illness. It is a mild program, but doing it with regularity is essential. If you have CFIDS, tailor the program to your specific tolerances. Your own good sense will dictate the amount of exercise that's healthiest for you.

As you can see, exercise really is the best remedy for chronic fatigue. It is a safe and effective self-help measure available to everyone, applicable to virtually every type of persistent tiredness. Your doctor can advise you as to whether there is any reason you should avoid the activity urged in this chapter. With his okay, you can start on the road to renewed energy right away.

CHAPTER

17

25 Hidden Causes of Fatigue (And Some Unexpected Cures)

Maybe it's true that a "rose is a rose is a rose," but fatigue is not fatigue is not fatigue. There are different types of fatigue and different ways to treat them. This is especially true of the kinds we'll consider in this chapter.

ALLERGIES SAP YOUR STRENGTH

If you have an allergy to something, you usually react to it with sneezing, reddened or watery eyes, rashes, difficulty breathing, poor sleep and fatigue. Fatigue can be one of the most troublesome symptoms of allergies and can be aggravated by the treatments commonly used.

In an allergic reaction, the body is mounting an immune response, fighting against an imagined enemy, in this case cat dander or ragweed pollen. The body mistakes these allergens for invaders such as deadly bacteria or viruses and defends against them in the same way. Therefore, just as fatigue is a common symptom of many infections, such as the influenza virus, it is present in most allergic conditions. The fatigue is a result of energy spent by the body in mounting an immune response.

Recent research has shown links between the fatigue of allergy and chronic fatigue immune dysfunction syndrome (CFIDS). In some studies, over half of the people who develop CFIDS have a history of multiple allergies or asthma. This tendency toward multiple allergies is seen as a genetic marker that identifies those who have an "overreactive," or hair-trigger, immune system. CFIDS can be considered an unusual immune response. But the unanswered question in CFIDS research is, an immune response to what?

Treatment that is normally effective in eliminating the fatigue of multiple allergies is less so in CFIDS. The standard treatment of allergies is desensitization shots. After determining what a person is allergic to, small doses of this substance are given by injection until the immune system grows tired of reacting to it and the allergy ceases. When this occurs, the symptoms of sneezing, itchy eyes, wheezing and fatigue usually disappear. Some allergy medications contain antihistamines, which get rid of the allergy symptoms but produce drowsiness as a by-product. If you suspect your allergy medication may cause fatigue for you, talk to your doctor about either a change in prescription or a smaller dose of your current medication to reduce the side effects.

A CURE FOR THE MIDWINTER ENERGY CRISIS

Some people say that being depressed has taken the light out of their lives. They mean this figuratively, of course. But a lack of sunlight can actually cause depression. And like other types of depression, it can lead to fatigue.

Seasonal affective disorder (SAD), a type of depression directly linked to a reduction in the amount of sunlight a person receives, is a well-known cause of chronic fatigue. SAD is most common in winter, obviously, and in polar regions where the nights are long. In its most ordinary form, SAD is the feeling of having the blues on a rainy day.

SAD is a biological problem that affects some of the basic body mechanisms involved in chronic fatigue. It can be treated effectively by exposing sufferers to bright lights for several hours a day and by increasing the person's exposure to natural sunlight.

Although no one knows exactly what causes SAD, research indicates that it is related to changes in brain chemistry and neurohormones. Norepinephrine, a chemical produced in the brain and linked to depression since the 1950s, is also involved.

THE CASE OF TOXIC ENERGY WASTE

Thomas thought that his constant fatigue was due to working two jobs. On his full-time job, he cleaned boiler vats at a chemical plant. That was at night. He also had a part-time day job.

Fatigue was his only problem—at first. Then, over a period of several months, Thomas developed memory problems, numbness of the arms and a skin rash.

Finally he was forced to take an extended sick leave, and he recovered completely. But as soon as he went back to work, the symptoms returned. First came the fatigue, then all the others quickly followed. Thomas chalked it up to the same problem as before—two jobs, working at night, not enough rest. But when an industrial toxicologist was consulted, he found that Thomas was suffering from chronic poisoning from the chemicals in the vats he was cleaning. The compounds were killing him!

Thomas changed jobs. He is no longer plagued by the failing memory, numbness or rash, and he is now fatigue free.

Another element believed to play a major role in SAD is melatonin, a hormone that is secreted at night as part of our biological clock's function. Melatonin helps us get tired enough to sleep.

But the same sunlight that can cure depression in some people can cause it in others. Those who suffer from reverse SAD get depressed in summer.

RX FOR SICK BUILDING SYNDROME

People who work in energy-efficient and well-sealed modern buildings are the ones most likely to develop sick building syndrome (SBS), a condition that is usually announced by dry or watery eyes, a stuffed-up nose, dry throat, nausea, dizziness, dry skin and fatigue.

A World Health Organization study showed that approximately 30 percent of all remodeled or new office buildings could serve as breeding grounds for SBS, and that between 10 and 30 percent of the people who work in those buildings will likely develop the condition. As a rule, SBS is caused by poor ventilation and circulation and is a by-product of energy conservation.

The most energy-efficient way to heat a building in the winter or cool it in the summer is to prevent as much of the treated air from escaping as possible. In other words, keep on circulating the treated air, no matter how contaminated it gets with smoke, the carbon dioxide we exhale, chemicals from the office equipment and furniture, paint fumes, the residue from industrial cleaning agents and so on. These pollutants build up and make people sick.

Going into the hospital to be treated or tested for the various conditions that SBS can cause may be no better than staying at work. A study in Sweden showed that hospital, health and social workers had the highest number of complaints about SBS.

The only real cure for SBS is to open a few windows or improve the ventilation so that the polluted air goes outside. Air filters might help, but not as much as letting in fresh air.

Pilots and flight crews who put in long hours flying at high altitudes in pressurized cabins can also suffer from a form of SBS caused by a combination of the chemicals in the plane, the air-conditioning system and the lack of fresh air. After all, you can't just open a window at 40,000 feet!

This can be a particular problem for flight attendants, since they are required to fly more often and therefore spend more time in the air than pilots and copilots do.

TAKE A BREAK FROM OVERTRAINING

Runners, take heed: A finely tuned high-performance race car is built to go fast—but not to go fast forever. If you run it too long and too hard beyond its limits, it will either blow up or burn out. The same thing can happen to your body.

One of the body's limiting factors is age. Another is lifestyle. Just because you could run five miles a day seven days a week when you were in college doesn't mean you can do it today and still do everything else that is expected of you. To prevent injury and what sports medicine experts call staleness, exercise physiologists suggest that sports enthusiasts limit their workouts to no more than five days a week. Also, to build your endurance without overdoing it, increase your mileage (if you run or bike) by no more than 10 percent a week.

If you work out on a regular basis and feel fatigued, cut back on exercise for a while. And get more sleep. If you're still tired in spite of taking a break from your exercise program, see your doctor. Once you start to regain energy, don't jump right back into the exercise routine that drained you in the first place.

Ease back into it slowly. Try some different exercises and some different activities. Vary your routine. If you used to run in the morning, try running in the evening. Don't let yourself go stale.

Exercise is probably the single best treatment for the fatigue of stress, depression, obesity and many other types of fatigue, but it can worsen the fatigue of CFIDS. Listen to your body. It will let you know if you are exercising too much or not enough.

And remember to increase your protein intake when you exercise. While carbohydrates may be the prime energy source during periods of exercise, fatigue follows if protein is used up and not replaced.

It's important to remember that anything can be harmful if taken to extremes. That includes exercise.

A PRESCRIPTION FOR COMMUTER FATIGUE

Spending an hour or so fighting traffic on your way to or from work is tiring. It's even worse if you spend the entire ride to work dwelling on everything that can go wrong and the ride home ruminating about what did (or did not) transpire.

Exhaust fumes, recycled air, the glare of the sun, traffic noise, potholes, an obnoxious radio talk-show host, tie-ups—these can drain even more energy.

If you have to commute, either as a driver or a passenger, here are tips on how to make the trip both more pleasant and more energizing.

Accept the fact that you are powerless over traffic. Accidents, traffic jams, delays, detours, flat tires and red lights happen. Take them in stride. Yours is just one car among thousands. You will get to your destination when you get there. Don't sweat it.

Travel in comfort. Would a back support make your trip more pleasant or prevent it from being painful? Then buy one. Do you want to listen to the radio? To a music cassette? How about a talking book? How about some silence? The choice is yours. If a cup of coffee or a can of soda makes the trip more enjoyable, indulge yourself. How about carrying a cooler stocked with some carrot sticks, grapes or fresh berries?

Passengers have rights, too. If the driver and person disagree on what to listen to, suggest that each person get a personal stereo—complete with headphones.

You're not at work until you're at work. Your trip is not work, so you needn't talk about your job or even think about it. To break the monotony, try different routes, or allow some time for side trips. Look at what goes on around you, and enjoy what you see. Turn the drive into an outing instead of a commute.

CONQUER COMPUTER FATIGUE

Sitting at a computer for hours at a time drains you. Your body gets tired from being in the same position for so long. Your eyes get tired from focusing on the screen. The fact that the temperature and humidity levels in some offices are designed for the computers instead of the humans who use them can just add to the discomfort. Here's how to make the best of it.

Get comfortable. Adjust the screen's distance from your eyes until it feels right. Make sure the keyboard is conveniently placed. Sit up straight. Don't hunch over. If you have a bad back, use a back support.

Take regular breaks. Get up and walk a bit. Move around in your seat to stretch your muscles.

Be good to your eyes. The human eye is most comfortable when it looks off into the distance. Staring at a computer screen requires the eye to contract its muscles, so when your eyes get tired, close them for a while, then look out a window. That lets the muscles relax. If you suffer from dry eyes, or if your eyes are sensitive to smoke and dust, conditions that can be aggravated by air-conditioning and recycled office-building air, ease the discomfort with artificial tears or eyedrops.

NIP BURNOUT IN THE BUD

When people are worn away by work or worry, we call it burnout. We usually talk about it in terms of jobs or careers, but burnout also strikes in relationships, hobbies or everyday struggles to survive. It's the product of months or years of almost constant stress and pressure that make your strength and energy gauges read "Empty." Then, like an overused oil lantern, you become only a burnt-out wick.

As a result, you're tired all the time and have a number of other health problems as well. Frequent colds, headaches, muscle aches and pains, upset stomach and digestion problems are the most common symptoms. And as a matter of fact, a report in *Behavioral Medicine* notes that burnout seems to overlap with CFIDS (a little-known observation). Common complaints among those who feel burned-out, tense or listless (or all three!):

- "I feel tired."
- "I feel physically exhausted."
- "I'm fed up."
- "My 'batteries' are dead."
- "I have no energy to go to work in the morning."

Others complain that they feel restless, mentally fatigued or sleepy.

We all get burned-out now and then for various periods. How long the burnout lasts, and how easily we recover from it, depends to a great extent on how far we let it go before we decide to do something about it. The key here is the decision to act.

It's easy to blame others for your situation—parents, kids, neighbors, co-workers . . . You could fill a book.

The truth is that you're probably not aware that you can take steps to prevent burnout. This doesn't mean you should quit your job, divorce your spouse or have your parents take over the care and feeding of your kids. It simply means you have to take care of yourself.

If you suffer from a case of work burnout, the odds are that you focus too much time—physical, mental and emotional time—on your work. If you only get away from the stress and pressure of work when you go home and immerse yourself in the stress and pressure of family life, you're really burning the candle at both ends. Your life is out of balance.

The only way to restore balance is to expand the other elements of your life or add new ones. Here are some tips for the "walking weary."

Call time-out. But don't limit your time-outs to a week or two a year, when you take a vacation, or one or two days a week. Sure, you need regular vacations, but you may also need regular daily breaks—from everything and everyone. Spend some time on yourself. And don't feel guilty! Instead of saying that you can't spare the time, ask yourself if you can afford a breakdown or maybe a stroke.

Do something different. Spend time doing something totally different from whatever is exhausting you. Get a hobby. Find things that you enjoy doing, and do them. If you are confined to a home or office and it feels as if the walls are going to crush you, get outside. If your day is spent in deafening noise, steal some quiet time. If you work with your brain, work out with your body, and vice versa.

If your job is burning you out and you see no relief in sight, you might want to consider asking for a lateral transfer to a different position. The new perspective may revitalize your energy (*and* productivity).

Examine what you do. Are your days' activities behind your burnout? Maybe it's less what you do than the way you do it, your attitude toward it, the people involved or how they act. Change your attitude or the way you operate and see if it makes a difference.

Check your priorities. Consider what burns you out and ask yourself one simple question: Is the activity really that important? Also ask who is most affected by what you're doing. Your boss? Your family? You?

Consider your motives. Why are you putting yourself through the aggravation, stress and misery? Do you really think it is that important? Do you want to impress someone? Are you trying to make someone look bad by comparison? Is it your aim to stay too busy to deal with other concerns? Many people use their jobs as an excuse to avoid their families; others use their families as an excuse to avoid taking care of business.

Check in with friends and family. Talk to people you love and respect about what you go through. Tell them what you do, why you do it and how it makes you feel. Pay attention to their replies and your feelings about them.

Don't do it alone. Refuse to take on the project by yourself. If someone dumps all the work on you, refuse to accept the entire load. If you're in charge, delegate some jobs. If no one else has any time for it, can it really be that important?

Eat, sleep and be merry. Make sure you eat well-balanced meals, get plenty of rest and put some fun into your life.

HOW TO DEAL WITH ROLE STRAIN

A variation of burnout fatigue is what psychologist Patricia Voydanoff has termed role strain—the pressure that comes from fulfilling the diverse roles of worker, spouse and parent, *simultaneously.*

Another psychologist, William J. Goode, says that the more roles we fill, the more strain we feel. But given the fact that wearing several different hats is a fact of contemporary life, there's not much you can do about shirking your bona fide responsibilities—showing up at your son's football game, satisfying your employer, spending time with your spouse, plus serving as household accountant, chauffeur, short-order cook, nurse, gardener, repair person, ad infinitum.

Here's what you can do, however, to relieve the weighty feeling that comes from role strain.

Consider the positive side of diversity. Psychologists contend that success in one area can take the sting out of failure in another. If you're a great seamstress, for example, you won't consider yourself a total failure if your last work assignment wasn't letter-perfect. People with a variety of selves handle criticism better.

Switch-hit. If you get bored with one role, you may get energized by stepping into another.

Take setbacks in stride. If you spread your energies around, a setback in any one area won't threaten your entire self-worth.

In short, psychologists report that if viewed positively, multiple roles are not a drain on energy but a *source* of energy. They enable you to handle ups and downs with less tension and anxiety.

A STRATEGY FOR SHIFT WORKER'S FATIGUE

Nearly a quarter of the American work force does shift work regularly, or at least occasionally. As a result, shift worker's fatigue is a major health problem in this country because it continually disrupts the worker's biological clock. This leads to chronic fatigue, sleep loss and difficulty with concentration and work performance.

As with jet lag, the basic problem is the inability to switch immediately from a day schedule to an afternoon, night or overnight schedule. Even though shift worker's fatigue can cost millions annually in poor performance and production as well as in injuries and accidents, many employers are only now beginning to treat it seriously.

Some shift workers adjust to rotating schedules easily, probably because of a more flexible biological clock. We all have our own circadian rhythms, which help determine our most productive periods. These rhythms can be sensed and measured by changes in bodily functions such as body temperature and the secretion of adrenal hormones, which helps the body get ready for sleep. Some of us are early birds, waking at dawn refreshed and ready to work; others are best late at night and hate to be active in the morning.

Those who have very flexible circadian rhythms and can quickly adjust to any schedule often lose this flexibility as they age. That's why elderly workers are much more likely to have shift fatigue. This is even true of people who have been working the same night shift for decades. As they get older, it gets harder.

But the circadian rhythm is only one factor. Perhaps even more important is the quality of life—or sleep—shift workers experience during their time off, especially if they try to operate on "normal" time on their days off.

Even permanent night workers constantly jump from their night schedule at work to a daytime schedule for their leisure, family and social activities. If their time-off social schedules matched their work schedules, there would be fewer problems. But it's hard to get a family or social life on that schedule—especially if you have children.

Chronic fatigue is almost inevitable for a night-shift worker who does not get enough sleep because of a full range of daytime activities. Still, shift work does not have to ruin your day—or your night. There are a number of remedies for shift worker's fatigue.

Employers and managers must also be made aware of the physical and mental problems shift work can cause. They must be able to identify warning signs in individual workers and be prepared to alter the schedule if there is any danger that a person's inability to cope with or adapt to shift work could cause an accident.

Some individuals—those who are naturally morning people, mothers with young children, the elderly and workers who lead an erratic lifestyle on their time off—are usually poor candidates for shift work. Employers must become more sensitive to the individual needs of their work force.

If you have shift worker's fatigue and are unable to change your schedule, concentrate on improving the quality of daytime sleep: Reduce noise, turn off the telephone, keep your bedroom as dark as possible, and guard against being awakened by children or friends.

Avoid changing your workday sleep patterns. Try to make your days off conform to the same sleep-and-wake schedule you follow on workdays. The more irregular the schedule, the greater the likelihood of chronic fatigue.

If you are on rotating shifts, it's easier to adjust if your shifts rotate toward "extending" the day—from nights to mornings, mornings to afternoons, afternoons to nights. As we'll see with jet lag, it is easier for the body to adjust to an extended day than to an abruptly shortened one.

GET A JUMP ON JET LAG

Whether you travel a couple of times a month or once in a blue moon, even a day or two of jet lag can seem like forever. No matter if it's for business or pleasure, the trip is probably important to you, and anything that interferes with it can be a major problem.

Jet lag would not be a problem if you traveled only within the same time zone—or if you could reset your body as easily as you reset your watch. But, of course, you can't.

Our bodies have set rhythms, known as circadian rhythms, which are set according to the clues our senses pick up around us. One of the most important of these rhythms is the sleep/wake cycle. Jet lag shows just how important it is.

Let's say you leave New York City at 5:00 P.M. and fly east to Europe, crossing numerous time zones in the process. Your body experiences a seven-hour flight. But when you arrive, the local time is completely different from what your body expects it to be. According to your body, it's midnight: "Go to sleep!" But a look at the nearest clock shows that it's 7:00 A.M.: "Wake up!"

In order to adjust, our bodies must undergo a phase shift, a biological shift from the nighttime rhythm to the daytime rhythm. This throws the biological clock into confusion, and we experience what is called jet lag: fatigue, sleepiness, headache, achiness, poor memory and concentration, and sometimes a feeling of disorientation and confusion. The symptoms last until the biological clock resets itself, perhaps after one day, two days or even a week. Often jet lag disappears just when you are ready to fly home, and then the process starts all over again.

The jet lag you experience after flying in one direction will be different from what you feel after flying the other way. It's worse when you fly east than when you fly west. Traveling east, from New York to Europe, the day is shortened, and for reasons still unknown, it is harder to resynchronize with a shortened day. Flying west lengthens the day. Our internal clock seems better able to manage to stretch a day than to shrink it.

Not every varied-time-zone traveler experiences jet lag; some people have very flexible circadian rhythms and adjust to a new time zone with barely a nap. But older people tend to suffer more from jet lag, probably because their biological clocks have become less flexible with the passage of years.

You can avoid or reduce jet lag by taking the following seven steps.

1. Stay calm while preparing for the trip. A frantic last-minute rush to pack and prepare, combined with a bumpy, noisy and cramped flight, causes more stress from jet lag than a relaxed departure.
2. Start to reset your biological clock before you leave. If, for example, you are flying east to Europe on Monday, begin changing on the Thursday before by going to bed early and waking up early—very early. If you are going west, start to stay up later a few days before departure. That way, when the time zones change, your biological clock will suffer less of a shock.
3. Reset your watch when you get on the plane. Being mentally adjusted to the new time zone makes it easier to get bodily adjusted. During the flight, try to eat and sleep as though you were already living in your destination's time zone.
4. Avoid alcohol during the flight. Drink tomato juice, club soda or orange juice instead.
5. Consider using medications. Over-the-counter antihistamines cause drowsiness and may help induce sleep on the plane. The rest you get tricks your biological clock into changing phases. Short-acting sedative-hypnotics or sleeping pills might accomplish the same thing without causing a hangover. The medications are intended for very-short-term

use only, just long enough to help the body adjust to the new timing of days and nights. One caveat, though: Don't borrow sleeping pills from a friend. See your doctor, so the type and dosage can be tailored to your needs.

6. Don't spend your first eight hours in bed after you arrive. If you arrive in the morning, take a short nap. Then go outside and let the daylight convince your body that it has to switch biological time zones. When it's dark out, the body produces a hormone called melatonin that causes drowsiness. Sunlight halts the production of the hormone, but indoor lighting won't do it. Go outside and take a walk. The walk will also help you relax after the trip.

7. Take it easy once you get there. Enjoy the trip, but don't overdo it during the first two or three days.

SOME BARRIERS FOR NOISE-RELATED FATIGUE

Noise is defined as loud and unwanted sound (usually made by something or someone else). Traffic, loud music, electronic equipment, machinery, aircraft, household appliances—the litany of familiar and annoying loud sounds could go on for pages. In truth, the world is getting noisier every day, and all that noise affects us. It has been linked to a number of medical and psychological conditions—stress, depression, irritability, high blood pressure, metabolism changes, gastrointestinal upsets, cardiovascular problems, ulcers—even fatigue.

It's not the noise itself that tires you, it's the stress and other reactions the noise can produce.

The best way to handle noise fatigue is to lower the volume on your life. Decorate your home with draperies, carpets, wall hangings and anything else that will absorb sound. Use sound-absorbing acoustic tiles on your ceilings, especially in noisy rooms. Place your washing machine, blender and other loud appliances on sound-absorbing rubber mats. Set limits on how loud the radio, stereo or TV can be played, and make sure that family members don't try to drown each other out.

Set aside some time every day to rest your ears, maybe by using a "white noise" machine or soothing background music to help block out traffic or neighborhood noises. Or you might want total silence.

As the noise level goes down in your life, your stress, depression and irritability levels do the same. Your blood pressure just might follow. Then your energy level can go up.

A NEW MIGRAINE MEDICINE

Migraine headaches can affect every waking moment of your day—and also the moments you could be sleeping. That's the main reason fatigue is often a major side effect of migraine headaches. The pain makes going to sleep difficult, if not impossible. Even for the lucky individuals who find they can sleep away a migraine, many find the aftermath leaves them drained and below par for a day or so.

What causes this particular type of headache? Migraines are due to changes in the size of the blood vessels in the brain. Usually the blood flow increases, causing the pounding sensation. This change in the blood flow affects the distribution of the blood in the brain and is believed to be responsible for other migraine symptoms, such as nausea, a tingling sensation and fatigue.

Oddly enough, migraines often develop while a person sleeps, particularly during the REM (rapid eye movement) or dreaming stages. Even though the headache pain might not wake you up, it prevents you from getting restful sleep.

Migraine headaches are virtually a field of medicine unto themselves. There are countless theories about why they happen and how they should be treated. Different remedies work for different people. In terms of fatigue, if you can bring your migraines under control, you should regain the energy those headaches steal from you. A promising new medicine, sumatriptan, offers hope for lifelong migraine sufferers and is worth asking your doctor about.

TAKE A HOLIDAY FROM DRINKING

Despite the initial lift it gives you, alcohol is a depressant. Its negative effect works on the brain, body and entire nervous system.

You get the early upper because the first thing alcohol depresses is your inhibitions. It just turns them off, reducing your worries and tensions and relaxing you. If you limit yourself to one or two drinks and don't indulge every day, you shouldn't have any problems.

But if you drink more, you court depression. The alcohol also slows down your reaction time and interferes with your ability to think, talk and move. If you're like a lot of people, after a few drinks you get tired, and all you want to do is lie down and go to sleep. If you drink too much, you pass out instead of actually sleeping. There is a difference, and you'll be painfully aware of it the next morning as you experience the exhaustion of a hangover (you know, that shaky, queasy, working-on-only-two-cylinders feeling that persists as you try to slog your way through the day after).

If you drink regularly—every day or several days a week—the alcohol and its side effects can build up in your body. It can take days or weeks to flush the accumulated alcohol completely out of your system.

The problems increase if you take alcohol with medications, especially tranquilizers (sedatives or sleeping pills) or antihistamines. It can also aggravate certain medical conditions such as ulcers, epilepsy, liver disorders *or chronic fatigue.*

If you drink regularly and wonder if it's causing or adding to your fatigue, give up alcohol for a while and see what happens. Switching to a fruit cooler, nonalcoholic beer or another less potent beverage could pay big dividends in renewed energy. If you can't stop drinking on your own, check into a recovery program or call Alcoholics Anonymous. You'll find AA and other recovery programs listed in the phone book.

If you're tired to start with and you want a drink that will pick you up, try ice water, coffee, tea, soda or fruit juice.

SMOKING DRAINS YOUR ENERGY, PUFF BY PUFF

Smokers who are accustomed to relying on nicotine for a lift several times a day may be surprised to learn that smoking actually reduces energy levels in several ways. The threat of cancer aside, smoking causes lung inflammation and destroys the elasticity of the lungs. As a result, the lungs lose their ability to absorb oxygen. As with heart disease, less oxygen means less energy.

Smoking also causes mucus to accumulate in the airways. This makes it harder for air to get through the air sacs and into the bloodstream. Further, smoking constricts the blood vessels, which causes poor blood circulation.

There's more. The carbon monoxide from cigarette smoke grabs hold and binds up the hemoglobin in blood cells, inhibiting the hemoglobin's ability to carry a full load of oxygen. The total effect is less oxygen in the tissues, which means less energy.

And the carbon monoxide is actually a poison. (If we measure a fire victim's carbon monoxide levels in the emergency room, we always ask if they smoke, since smokers normally show a much higher carbon monoxide level than nonsmokers.)

In younger people with otherwise healthy hearts and lungs, smoke-related fatigue is relatively slight—at first—because their systems can compensate for the lost oxygen. But as people get older and more tissue is damaged, the effects become more pronounced and longer lasting.

If you suffer from some other fatigue-causing condition, smoking will just make it worse. For example, if you have sleep-based chronic fatigue or any sleep disorder, smoking can aggravate it. Smoking can even cause sleep disorders by increasing the amount of obstruction in the nasal passages.

Medical studies show that the main reason people smoke is to relieve stress. In stressful situations, people light up more frequently. And the anger, mood swings and even rage that occur when smokers quit are infamous. This is especially true in individuals who light up when they're nervous and use nicotine as a sedative. While nicotine may calm emotions momentarily, it creates an addiction that is notoriously difficult to break. In this way, the stress perpetuates the smoking habit. So dealing with stress is one way to escape smoker's fatigue.

In another intriguing bit of news, a study presented to the American Psychiatric Association by Naomi Breslau, Ph.D., reported a link between smoking and depression, a common cause of fatigue. Dr. Breslau suspects that nicotine dependence is somehow related to major depression. Dr. Breslau, director of research in the psychiatry department at Henry Ford Hospital in Detroit, theorizes that there may be some long-term effect of nicotine dependence that researchers have yet to uncover.

If you want to determine the effect of smoking on your energy levels, try this test: Go several hours without a cigarette (which should be easy enough to do, given the ongoing increase in smoking restrictions in the workplace and public buildings). Then light up as usual. About one minute after finishing this cigarette, you will

THE CASE OF THE OVERENERGIZED COLLEGE STUDENT

During a visit with a friend one Saturday night, David was introduced to a new computer game that featured jet fighters, bombs, guns and missiles, plus lots of explosions and noise. It required great coordination, intense concentration, instantaneous reactions and a high degree of digital dexterity.

David spent an hour getting warmed up and passing through the first level of enemy fighters. After the third cup of coffee, he had the hang of it and his reflexes were razor sharp.

David played for another six hours while he went through a six-pack of cola (sweetened with sugar) and enough junk food to satisfy a roomful of ravenous teenagers. He beat the game, killing off all the enemies and saving the world. When David realized he had been playing for seven hours, he was stunned. To him it had felt like 15 minutes.

He was tired, but totally exhilarated.

Thirty minutes later he almost fell apart. He had never felt so wiped out in his life. At 4:00 A.M. he drove home in a daze, then slept for eight hours.

Although he had not had any alcohol, David woke up with a hangover, still exhausted. He was also nervous and jittery.

He had been overstimulated. The caffeine, coupled with seven hours of playing a mesmerizing computer game that required complete concentration, had drained him. It took him a week to regain his normal energy.

experience a wave of fatigue that lasts about five minutes. Many smokers describe this wave of exhaustion as feeling like "a plug had been pulled."

With chronic cigarette use, this fatigue is spread out more evenly and is less noticeable. If you are a smoker, watch your energy level for ten minutes after the first cigarette in the morning. If you really want to become fatigue free, this experience may be more convincing in getting you to quit than the medical studies on heart disease and lung cancer!

Speaking of which: Smokers with heart disease do not complain much about fatigue, even though it may be severe. The reason is that they know why the fatigue is there, and they also know that their disease may be fatal. One of the saddest ironies is that it's much easier to quit smoking once you develop heart disease and know that if you don't, you will die.

COFFEE DRINKER'S FATIGUE

Generally we don't think of caffeine as something that makes you tired. We think of it as relief from tiredness, providing that needed jolt of energy for waking up or staying alert. Caffeine does do that—up to a point.

Caffeine, by the way, is all around us, not only in coffee, tea, soft drinks, cocoa and chocolate, but also in prescriptions and over-the-counter pain relievers, diuretics, cold remedies and weight-control pills.

In some ways caffeine acts like sugar. Sugar generates energy; caffeine generates adrenaline (the action hormone from the adrenal gland). In both cases the initial high is followed by a low. With sugar, the slump comes when the immediate source of energy is used up. With caffeine, the low occurs when the adrenaline is used up.

Like sugar, caffeine also depletes the B vitamins stored in the body.

Because caffeine is a stimulant, large doses can excite you enough to make you tense and anxious as well as sleepless. It also acts as a diuretic, increases the heart rate and can cause heart irregularities. Some researchers believe that heavy caffeine users are more prone to coronary disease than others, although this has yet to be proven.

On the plus side, along with the short-term lift it gives you, caffeine decreases blood flow to the brain. This helps in treating some types of migraine headaches, which also leave people drained and listless.

Depending upon what you drink and the way it is made, you could be getting a lot more caffeine than you think. The real question is, are you getting too much?

Some of us are convinced that we'd collapse at our desk without our morning cup of coffee or tea. But today many people are learning that they can shake the caffeine habit and have even more energy.

True, withdrawal could involve several days or even a week of minor discomfort and, in some cases, headaches, but these soon disappear along with caffeine-induced nervousness, tension and jumpiness.

Most of us get our caffeine from coffee, the world's most valuable legal agricultural commodity. People in the United States alone drink more than $4 billion worth every year, about 20 percent of it as instant coffee.

Your morning cup can provide 30 to 175 milligrams of caffeine, depending on the type of coffee itself, the beans it was brewed from, how it was brewed and—of course—the size of your mug. That's why the number of cups you drink doesn't always reflect the amount of caffeine you take in.

A cup of drip coffee contains more caffeine than the same amount of percolated. That's because in drip coffeemakers, the water passes through the filter only once, so more coffee is needed. In a percolator, the water keeps circulating through the same coffee, so less is needed. Caffeine is absorbed by the hot water as it passes over the grounds, so the more coffee there is in the pot, the more caffeine there is to be absorbed.

Instant coffee, which is prebrewed, has less caffeine than the other types. To manufacture instant coffee, extremely thick, almost syrupy liquid is forced through an atomizer, and the mist is then sprayed through a jet of hot air. The hot air evaporates the water in the extract, and the remaining dried coffee particles are then packaged.

Freeze-dried coffee also starts as a thick syrup, which is frozen and put into a vacuum that extracts the water; the residue is packaged.

Naturally decaffeinated coffee is lowest in caffeine. To make it, the green coffee bean is processed in a steam or chemical bath that removes the caffeine.

FATIGUE FROM COFFEE'S COUSINS

Even if you're not hooked on coffee, you can experience caffeine-related fatigue.

Tea has less caffeine than coffee—10 to 100 milligrams a cup, depending on the type and amount of leaves used, how long the tea steeps and the size of the cup.

While boiling water absorbs caffeine from coffee almost immediately, getting the caffeine out of tea leaves takes longer. So the longer the tea steeps, and the more tea you have in the pot, the more caffeine you will have.

There are various caffeine-free herbal teas on the market, but read the labels carefully before you buy. Just because a tea is called raspberry, orange spice or some other innocent-sounding name and claims to have all natural ingredients, that does not mean it is caffeine free. Flavorings are sometimes mixed with regular tea, and the result is just a tea of a different color and taste, not a caffeine-free brew.

The real fizz in soft drinks. Most caffeinated soft drinks contain between 40 and 50 milligrams of caffeine in a 12-ounce serving, and over 95 percent of that is added during processing. In most regular cola-type drinks, the remaining 5 percent comes from kola nuts. In fact, Coca-Cola, created in the 1880s as the first cola drink, took its name from the kola nut that provides much of its flavor. Most dark-colored soft drinks contain caffeine, with the exception of root beer.

Today there is a growing demand for caffeine-free soft drinks. Many people find that, once they get used to drinking caffeine-free colas, they cannot taste a difference.

By the way, a diet version of a brand-name soft drink usually contains the same amount of caffeine as the regular version.

The secret of chocolate and cocoa. The sweeter and darker the chocolate, the more caffeine it has. A standard chocolate bar usually contains about 10 milligrams; a cup of hot cocoa or chocolate milk has less than that. Cocoa and chocolate also contain a chemical called theobromine, which has an effect similar to that of caffeine.

MEDICINE CABINET FATIGUE

Any drug you take can raise or lower your energy levels. Monitor how you're affected and remember that even if it's a stimulant, you will come down eventually.

If you take an over-the-counter drug, read the package insert to see if the medication can cause fatigue. In the case of prescription drugs, ask your pharmacist about any side effects that might affect your energy and about the combined effects of mixing various drugs.

Talk to your doctor before you stop taking any prescribed medication. If your physician says you don't need it, but you can't stop or taper off on your own under medical supervision, check into a recovery program or call Narcotics Anonymous. They can help you with addiction to either prescription or street drugs. You'll find recovery programs and Narcotics Anonymous listed in the phone book.

BREAK THE NIGHTTIME EATING SYNDROME

This odd clue to fatigue is another example of a cluster of symptoms that may be classified in many different categories. It's an eating disorder, a sleep disorder and a stress-related disorder. It also causes chronic fatigue and is characterized by excessive eating at night combined with the inability to eat in the morning.

After a nighttime eating binge, the individual is unable to sleep, tossing and turning for hours, interspersed with more eating. Obesity is a common (and predictable) consequence of this syndrome, but severe fatigue also results, probably from the insomnia.

It is commonly accepted that both the eating and the insomnia are individual reactions to stress and that stress disorders are at the root of the symptoms. The best treatment is a combination of counseling, stress reduction and improved dietary habits.

PERFECTIONISM-INDUCED WEARINESS

A lot of people feel compelled to be perfect. If they aren't perfect, they feel they aren't any good at all. Think of the third-grader who obsesses over the single spelling word he got wrong instead of celebrating the 99 he got right.

Feeling the need to do everything perfectly wastes a lot of time and effort. Perfectionists can put as much into wrapping the garbage as they do into wrapping a birthday present. That might be a slight exaggeration, but when you go into everything with that attitude, you get tired often.

Perfectionism also produces a lot of stress and pressure and can lead to burnout, which we looked at earlier.

If perfectionism is your problem, here are several principles that can help you to overcome it.

No one is perfect. Accept the fact that you are not and never will be perfect, and that you don't have to be perfect to be loved and valued.

Give yourself permission to make mistakes. If you aren't willing to make mistakes, you aren't willing to learn and grow.

Try one new thing every day. You'll make mistakes, but you'll be a better person for the experience.

Some jobs don't need to be done perfectly. If you're submitting a book to a publisher, spend a lot of time checking your spelling, punctuation and grammar. If you're posting an appointment reminder on the refrigerator, make sure the time and date are correct; the spelling and penmanship only need to be close.

There's a difference between a mistake and a failure. Playing the wrong notes on the piano is making a mistake. Refusing to play the piano because you're afraid of hitting the wrong keys makes the incident a failure.

Practice not being perfect. Look at something you obsess over and force yourself to do it less than perfectly. If you can't stand a thing out of place in the house, for instance, clean the house and leave a single dustball in the middle of the floor; leave it there for several days. If the excuse note you write to your child's teacher has a mistake, scratch it out instead of rewriting the entire note. Use your imagination to break your perfection habits.

MANAGING MITRAL VALVE PROLAPSE

When someone experiences fatigue, chest pain and heart palpitations, the first thought is usually "I'm having a heart attack!" Yet this cluster of symptoms is very common to a condition known as mitral valve prolapse.

The mitral valve governs an opening between two of the heart's four chambers, ensuring that blood will travel in only one direction through the heart. Sometimes the valve can be floppy or loose, and with back pressure it can bulge, or "prolapse." Specific tests can visualize this valve, and too large a bulge signals mitral valve prolapse.

Some estimates say that up to 30 percent of young women have a floppy mitral valve, although the vast majority have no medical problems with it. In these individuals the trivial prolapse is a variation of normal and of no consequence. In others, however, the floppy mitral valve is related to an irregular heartbeat, episodes of shortness of breath and fatigue, and these people are said to have "mitral valve prolapse syndrome." While it is usually not dangerous, mitral valve prolapse is uncomfortable and frightening for the victim.

Not many long-term studies have been done on the course of this illness. However, few authorities believe that mitral valve prolapse will lead to any significant heart disease, and the condition may actually improve over time. Debate exists over the relationship between mitral valve prolapse syndrome and CFIDS, as it is very common in CFIDS to have palpitations and shortness of breath. Is it possible that an underlying condition, CFIDS, could cause both the floppiness of the valve and the palpitations? The matter has not been resolved.

The irregular heartbeat or chest discomfort is rarely dangerous, but it should always be checked by a physician. Other conditions, such as rheumatic heart disease, can cause hardening of the mitral valve, and this is a form of heart disease that requires careful monitoring by a physician. Rheumatic disease of the mitral valve is easily separated from mitral valve prolapse by testing. The condition can be dangerous and should not be overlooked. Certain other forms of mitral valve disease, particularly in persons with curvature of the spine, also need careful monitoring.

Good remedies for mitral valve prolapse are available. Medications (beta blockers or calcium channel blockers) can eliminate the palpitations and slow the heart rate. The fatigue is not so easy to treat, particularly since these same medications may cause fatigue. While medical studies are not conclusive, exercise may improve the condition by decreasing the levels of the adrenal hormones that worsen the palpitations. But as with any heart condition, exercise should be carefully monitored by a physician.

FIBROMYALGIA, A COUSIN OF CFIDS

Many people consult a doctor because of aching muscles, joint pain, weakness and fatigue, only to learn that they suffer from fibromyalgia, once called fibrositis. *Fibromyalgia* literally means "pain in the muscles." The prominent joint or muscle pain of this condition is different from rheumatoid arthritis or lupus erythematosis. The cause is unknown, but it's probably neither emotions nor depression.

The difference between fibromyalgia and other forms of arthritis is mainly that the joints do not become hot or swollen, and blood tests for arthritis are negative. Yet the pain can be almost as severe, and medical studies show that the degree of disability can be nearly as great as in arthritis. Some studies hint that there is muscle damage in fibromyalgia, as measured by elevated muscle enzymes after exercise.

A growing school of thought says fibromyalgia is the same condition as CFIDS, as sleep disturbance, headache, memory and concentration problems and abdominal distress are also a part of fibromyalgia. There is no clear difference between CFIDS and fibromyalgia in children, and either term may be used to describe this symptom pattern. It is likely that the term "fibromyalgia" is more commonly used when muscle pain is the most severe symptom, and "CFIDS" is used when fatigue is the most severe symptom. Both illnesses have a similar favorable long-term outlook. I believe that, in time, research will show fibromyalgia and CFIDS are actually the same illness.

Treatment for the condition is usually based on the use of nonnarcotic medications that reduce pain, such as aspirin or acetaminophen, similar to the treatment of arthritis. The use of tricyclic antidepressants has also been found to reduce the pain. One of the leading muscle relaxants, cyclobenzaprine, is a drug of this class. Exercise is generally recommended, although some persons with fibromyalgia will have a worsening of fatigue and muscle pain, similar to that seen with CFIDS. (See chapter 16.)

POOPED BY PMS

The inner tension called premenstrual syndrome (PMS) that some women feel just before their period begins can include a variety of different mental, physical and emotional symptoms, including irritability, depression, headaches, fatigue, puffiness and pain in the breasts.

The condition appears to be based on hormonal and fluid changes and water retention, and the difficulty of adjusting to these physical changes. Strictly speaking, PMS is not a disease or an illness. It is a perfectly natural—though unpleasant—condition.

As with many other types of fatigue, once the other symptoms are dealt with, the tiredness usually disappears on its own. Medical treatment aimed at evening out hormonal changes may improve

PMS symptoms, but results vary. Individual patients respond differently to commonly employed measures that include reducing caffeine intake, eating fewer sweets and getting more exercise. Some physicians find hormone therapy effective. (Birth control pills are a familiar prescription for PMS.)

PREGNANCY PLAYS YOU OUT

While neither pregnancy nor breast-feeding is an illness or a disease, both can trigger marked slumps in a normally active woman's energy levels. To begin with, a pregnant woman actually does eat for two (or more), so her energy (that is, calorie) needs go way up.

When a woman is pregnant, her blood circulation is reduced. That's because blood is temporarily shunted to the growing fetus, away from other parts of the mother's body. Her metabolism is altered, too.

With the increase in girth, a pregnant woman's center of gravity shifts so it's harder for her to get up from a bed or a chair. Hormonal changes that can cause varying emotions occur commonly during pregnancy and contribute to the increased fatigue. She is also more susceptible to mood swings, depression, stress and other emotional states that take the starch out of mind and body.

Complicating matters is the fact that while the expectant mother needs more sleep, sleep patterns are also different during pregnancy. In early pregnancy, women tend to feel generalized fatigue and sleep longer. In the second three months of pregnancy, the sleep period returns to normal despite the fatigue, but in the last three months, pregnant women tend to develop insomnia and difficulty sleeping.

Sleep studies conducted during the last three months show disordered sleep stages. Most sleep specialists feel that the insomnia is due entirely to physical discomfort. It is common for women to continue with sleep disturbances after delivery, gradually returning to their prepregnancy pattern.

But even though the woman's body may be ready to resume normal nighttime sleep, a new baby might have other plans for that time and remind her of them often in the middle of every night.

As with pregnancy, the emotional demands of breast-feeding can be almost as draining as the physical demands. Therefore, a nursing woman also requires more energy and more sleep.

There's really no mystery to coping with the fatigue of pregnancy. Setting priorities helps. You may find that now that you're producing a child, other tasks—like getting all your errands done on time, taking on extra projects at work or entertaining at home—have to be postponed or delegated. Taking frequent short naps, avoiding caffeine and doing stretching exercises may be helpful (even advisable). The key is to remember that although you may be sitting stock-still, your body is working feverishly to create a wonderful new human being. So you're not "wasting" time!

And by the way, pregnancy is one type of fatigue that is definitely contagious, since many new fathers suffer from it, too.

PUTTING ZIP INTO MENOPAUSE

Menopause signals a change in a woman's life that occurs when the ovaries cease to function and the body's estrogen content falls. The ensuing imbalance in female hormones causes the symptoms of menopause (hot flashes, fatigue, irritability, insomnia, chills, sweats and dry skin). Up to 20 percent of women have little or no difficulty with menopause and merely notice the absence of the monthly menstrual cycle. For another 20 percent, the symptoms may be very unpleasant, significantly disrupting their lives. The group of women between these extremes will notice the symptoms to varying degrees.

The most dramatic symptoms of menopause are usually hot flashes along with vaginal dryness. Both are directly attributable to a lack of estrogen. Treatment with estrogen replacement therapy (ERT) usually removes these symptoms and improves many of the others.

ERT is controversial among physicians. While estrogen replacement may improve symptoms, it does not eliminate menopause, it merely delays it. On the plus side is the possible prevention of heart attacks and osteoporosis—thinning of the bones, which makes them weaker and prone to fractures. On the negative side are the reports that estrogen replacement may increase the risk of uterine cancer and foster the growth of certain breast cancers. These two concerns have been addressed by lowering the estrogen dose in therapy to where it is still effective in removing the symptoms of menopause but lowers the risks.

The fatigue of menopause (like most conditions causing fatigue) has several components. Perhaps the most important cause, and the easiest to treat, is sleep disturbance due to hot flashes. Menopausal women may wake up numerous times during the night with hot flashes and sometimes drenching sweats, and the disturbed sleep translates to fatigue. ERT eliminates the hot flashes, sweats and sleep disturbance, usually with ease.

The emotional changes include mood swings or irritability that may accompany the estrogen loss at menopause. While uncomfortable, these mood changes may fluctuate from hour to hour but seldom cause life disruption. They can be improved by ERT.

Sometimes the fatigue is related to depression or changes in the emotions, as menopause may be an important symbol of lost youth, missed chances and changes in activities or interests. In this regard, the fatigue of menopause blends into retirement fatigue as depression takes hold. Usually our life changes occur so slowly that we do not appreciate them. Only when some symbol (such as menopause) crystallizes the passage of time do we fully understand the implications of our growing and developing. But like retirement, menopause may signal a great new era in a woman's life. Rather than regret a lost adolescence, she can make changes in her life based on wisdom and experience. The fatigue of loss can be replaced by the enthusiasm of change.

The debate concerning menopause and its treatment by ERT has been vocal. Proponents state that the reduction of symptoms and improved lifestyle is great, while the risks are small. Opponents argue that any increased risk is unacceptable. My feeling is that the woman undergoing menopause should be able to make the choice without difficulty, given accurate information by her physician. If her life is truly unpleasant because of the symptoms, ERT is quite reasonable. The possibility of treatment with estrogen to prevent osteoporosis should be discussed with a physician.

BEATING THE RETIREMENT DOLDRUMS

Strictly speaking, the fatigue often associated with retirement is a form of depression. After many years of a clearly defined work activity, many people who face retirement are at a loss for how to fill their time. Retirement may be associated with advancing age, becoming useless, even approaching death. For many of us, our work defines who we are, and our productivity proves our worth. So some equate retirement with uselessness, the basis of depression.

Fortunately, our society is changing and retirement is less automatic for people who remain good at their work and wish to continue. Being old is not strictly defined by the years that have passed, and society is beginning to appreciate the wisdom and experience that can come with 30 years on a job.

Those who look forward to retirement are unlikely to experience retirement fatigue. They have dreams of traveling, doing volunteer or community work or getting on with a hobby. For them, retirement is not filled with "make-work" but is a genuine opportunity to do things they have always longed to do.

In planning for retirement, assess your own psychological state. If you are the kind of person who needs to be active, busy and productive to feel good about yourself, plan your retirement to fit those needs. Be realistic about your health, but fill your time with the long-dreamed-of activities. Prepare for your retirement before "falling" into it. Try out different things. Decide if traveling is for you and what sorts of pastimes you might enjoy. Before you actually find yourself in retirement, consider your family needs and explore ideas of what you would really like to do.

On the other hand, if you are the person who has dreamed of relaxing, of finally getting the chance to rest after running around for the past 30 or 40 years, do it and enjoy. Don't make up activities just because you think you should. If you want to retire . . . retire!

PART III

THE 30-DAY HIGH-ENERGY PROGRAM

Positive Steps You Can Take to End Fatigue

This section consists solely of a comprehensive 30-day plan to combat fatigue. By now you've probably identified the major factors that feed your fatigue, and you can use that information to maximize the benefits you derive from this program. Since any kind of fatigue—chronic fatigue immune dysfunction syndrome (CFIDS) in particular—has many components, this program addresses *all* possible factors: physical, mental, emotional and spiritual.

You must prepare for this program, just as you would for any important undertaking. It isn't something to begin casually on a random day. At the very least, you'll want to scan the daily instructions to prepare for certain tasks.

The first week might be a little tough. But as you persevere, you'll begin to feel significant improvement. Then the renewed enthusiasm and mood elevations that follow will breed further improvement, and the subsequent weeks will fly by. Concentrate on consistency and determination.

Part of the program consists of spiritual advice and practices like meditation. I've found that people who pay attention to their spiritual side do better in life than others. Perhaps it reduces depression or cuts back on the actual degree of disability and discomfort. Many experts believe that spirituality affects a person's ability to cope. Any and all of those possibilities make spirituality an important part of this program, regardless of your particular denomination or belief system.

One caution: If you are seriously depressed, skip the suggestions on meditation beginning on Day 19. Psychologists have found that, in general, depressed patients tend to do better if they focus their attention outward, rather than within themselves. If you feel depressed, just do the suggested exercises and other nonreflective activities.

FIRST, CHECK IN WITH YOUR DOCTOR

Before you embark on this program, it's a good idea to have a complete physical examination done. There are a number of things you want to know: What is the most likely cause of your fatigue? Do you have any medical conditions, such as high blood pressure or diabetes, that might require modifications in your activity or diet? Does your doctor have any ideas about what might work best for you? (The opening chapters of this book cover a wide range of often-overlooked causes of fatigue, plus appropriate solutions.)

If you've been diagnosed with a specific medical condition, your doctor may prescribe a special diet for you. If so, follow his or her advice in place of the nutritional suggestions in our program. (For example, if you've been diagnosed with an undereating disorder—a clear threat to energy levels—the suggestions for cutting fat and calories from your diet probably won't apply.)

Your doctor will most likely order a few blood tests to measure your hemoglobin, cholesterol, triglycerides and so forth. Ask for the results, then enter these levels in your fatigue diary, described below. That way, as you proceed with your program and make improvements in your diet and exercise habits, you'll have a benchmark to help you monitor your progress.

Naturally, you'll want to ask if your doctor condones a mild exercise program for you, in light of your physical exam. Chances are your physician will be fairly supportive. If he or she suggests a specific regimen—say, for arthritis or some other medical condition—substitute that for the program suggested here.

Also be sure to ask about any medications you may be taking, especially if you've been relying on sleeping pills, antidepressants or any other drugs customarily prescribed for insomnia, tension and so forth. One of the goals of this program is to minimize reliance on these types of medications, so you'll want to follow your doctor's advice regarding dosages.

IF YOU SMOKE, QUIT

Because smoke compromises the oxygen-extracting power of your lungs and pollutes your bloodstream with energy-draining poisons, giving up smoking (including cigars and pipes) is an essential part of any energy-enhancing program.

If you don't smoke, you're already ahead of the game. Otherwise it's essential to quit, for reasons explained in chapter 17. Not everyone can quit cold turkey, of course. Here again, your physician may be able to advise you on what method is best for you—nicotine patches, nasal sprays, smoking-cessation programs or a combination of methods. This will enable you to stop with minimal difficulty. But be determined! The damaging effects of this single factor on your health are alarming.

THE FATIGUE DIARY

This is an essential part of the 30-day program. It will amount to a written record of the events and thoughts of the month, and it will help you to focus on the issues that are most important regarding your specific fatigue. First, grade your energy level on a scale of 0 (no energy) to 10 (full of vitality). Then, throughout the program, you'll find instructions on what to cover in your diary: stress, emotions, exercise, nutrition, sleep—anything that might have a bearing on your fatigue.

Each day kicks off with an affirmation to help you institute one of the steps for that day, followed by stress-reduction tips, "emotional calisthenics," exercise guidelines and tips for either jettisoning energy-draining foods or adding vitality-boosting nutrients to your diet. And if poor sleep has been throwing a monkey wrench into your generators, you'll find step-by-step tips for getting a good night's sleep every night.

Later you will probably want to reflect on the factors that were most helpful to you. In a way, the diary is your psychotherapist; when you write things down, matters become clearer, just as they would if you were confiding in a therapist or trusted friend.

Your diary is personal and private, for your eyes only, so don't be embarrassed about its contents. Write anything you want, but be honest with yourself. After 30 days, it will show you how far you've come!

TAKE YOUR TIME

If you need more time, go slowly. The suggestions are generally appropriate for persons with CFIDS as well as for those with mild to moderate fatigue. However, if you suffer severe fatigue, as with CFIDS, it might be best to proceed at a less ambitious pace. Given the individualized nature of this illness, you may need to select only those exercises and tips that apply to you, or modify them to match your goals and energy levels.

Either way, take these steps at your own pace. Thirty days is an ideal, but if it takes you 60 days—or 90, or longer—to work through the program, so be it. Given the fact that many people suffer from low energy levels for years without hope, two or three months is still a very short recovery time!

DAY 1

Affirmation

Today is not just the first day of the rest of my life, it is the beginning of a new way of life. I will mark this great new beginning by starting a daily journal of my thoughts.

Stress Reduction

Take 15 minutes today to think about what upsets you on a day-to-day basis, and describe your feelings in your diary. Of course, merely naming various demands or annoyances doesn't mean you can or will eliminate the pressure they exert. Raising three children, for example, can certainly be taxing (and usually is). But since it's too late to abstain from parenthood, your only alternative is to learn how to cope with it better.

And so it is with any stress. For now simply make a note of whatever stresses are affecting you. Don't make any effort to eliminate them today. Be an impartial observer of your own life. Record accurately what you see. You cannot begin to fight against stress until you recognize what it is and what causes it. These two elements—detached observation and acknowledgment—will help you prepare for the attack.

Emotions

Think about any single mistake you made in the past two months that weighs heavily upon you. Forgive yourself for that mistake, and move on.

Nutrition

Today focus on your typical daily diet. Eat what you normally do. Then, for the next five days, record everything you eat and drink in your fatigue diary.

There's no need to weigh every serving or count calories or grams of fat (unless you're already doing so as part of a weight-loss program). But do make note of the portions you eat—a cone of ice cream or a bowlful, for example. A bag of chips or a handful. One slice of pizza or the whole pie.

For easy reference, it's best to devote a separate page of your diary to your food-intake record. For example:

Breakfast: Two scrambled eggs, two pieces of toasted white bread, a glass of orange juice, two cups of coffee with sugar.

Midmorning snack: A sticky bun, one cup of coffee with sugar.

Lunch: A tuna sandwich on white bread, a glass of milk, an orange.

Snack: A can of cola.

Dinner: Two pieces of chicken, mashed potatoes with butter, steamed carrots, apple pie, a glass of milk, two cups of coffee.

Snack: Half a bag of corn chips, two beers.

The point of this exercise is to examine the pattern of your typical diet to see if it is heavy on sweets, fat, caffeine and so on. You will refer back to this nutrition part of the fatigue diary often during the rest of the month. For the program to work, you need to be honest with yourself.

Sleep

If you do not take sleeping medications now, you can skip this part. But many people rely on sleeping pills (benzodiazepines) in a near-desperate attempt to get more sleep and obliterate daytime fatigue. For simple insomnia (that is, not related to a major, temporary upheaval in life, such as the death of a spouse), chronic use of sleeping pills only worsens sleep over time. So one goal of the 30-day program is to wean you off them slowly.

As mentioned in the discussion of the physical exam, if you are on sleeping pills, it is essential that you ask your physician if it is safe to try a period without them. Some medical conditions might lead your physician to recommend against this, and you should follow that advice. But if your physician encourages you to cut back (and chances are he or she will), review these guidelines together. If you want to cut back on your medications at a different pace, it is generally safe to do so. (It will be harder for you at first if you speed your break from the pills, but you'll be rid of them that much sooner.)

Either way, the first week of decreasing sleeping medications may prove difficult. It's very easy to develop a tolerance to these medications—that is, your body may have forgotten how to fall asleep without assistance—and at first your insomnia may become worse before it improves. But hang in there; it *will* improve.

On the first night decrease your dose of sleeping medication by half and maintain this dose for five days. Most medications are scored so that dividing a tablet in half is simple. Otherwise you may have to ask your physician to rewrite your prescription to reflect the lower dose.

DAY 2

Affirmation

I will find some quiet time today and spend it thinking about everything good in my life and becoming more aware of the wonderful ways each thing affects me.

Stress Reduction

Review yesterday's entry. You may have listed 20 or 30 different stresses in your life. Now rewrite the list in order of which cause you the most anguish and discomfort. Your list, for example, might start with "1. The one-hour drive to work and back" and end with "18. I owe my old college roommate a letter."

Make note of any additional stresses that have occurred to you since yesterday. Most people find that once they start looking for stresses, more and more of them become obvious.

Don't try to change anything yet—you're still in the process of building awareness. You may notice, however, that once you see some of these stresses for what they really are—trivial annoyances—the minor ones begin to disappear on their own.

Emotions

Think about any insult or slight you may have received in the past month, perhaps from a friend, perhaps from a business associate. Forgive that person for the offense. Just let it go and move on. Enjoy the lightness and energy that comes from jettisoning negative feelings of resentment and hurt.

Nutrition

Enter your nutrition notes for Day 2 of your fatigue diary. Pay special attention to your caffeine intake. Beginning today, try to steadily reduce the amount of caffeine you consume. Remember, a can of soda has about the same amount as half a cup of coffee. And those super-jumbo-colossal cups of soda at convenience stores have even more.

Start by eliminating caffeine after 5:00 P.M. Have your normal amount during the day. Continue this until Day 8. (Of course, if you already limit your caffeine intake to the first ten waking hours of the day, you don't have to worry about this for now.)

Sleep

Note what time you go to bed. The next day, try to estimate how long it took you to fall asleep and the total number of hours you slept. Also make a note of any naps you took—at what time and how long you slept.

DAY 3

Affirmation

I don't have to eliminate stress today, but I will pay attention to how my body reacts to pressure and learn how it affects me. That way I can begin to use the best in me to reduce worrying.

Look for the sweaty palms, nervous chatter, gritted teeth, racing heartbeat. When you can recognize the signs of stress in yourself, you can begin to eliminate that stress.

Stress Reduction

Review your list of stresses from Day 1 and choose the five that are least meaningful in your life. These are the ones you will try to eliminate first.

Unfortunately, we cannot get rid of all stress in life. Life is basically one big stress. But not all stresses are necessary. The kids and the job are stressful, but they're hardly unnecessary. But how about the stress of having to bake a pie for next week's office party? Put it near the top of the list of "eliminate-ables." After all, you can always stop at a bakery and *buy* a pie.

It would be nice if the totally unnecessary and avoidable stresses were at the top of your list, but it's more likely that they are toward the bottom. That's okay. Once you have some success eliminating the unnecessary stresses, you gain the courage to tackle the more difficult ones.

Emotions

Try to remember a book you've read, a sermon, lecture or speech you've heard or a movie you've seen that was meaningful for you, one that inspired you and gave you a lift for the day. If you still have the book, page through it. Or mentally review the highlights of the talk. Or rent a videotape of the movie and watch it again. If possible, time this activity for the early evening, so you can allow the glow of your emotions to take over the rest of the evening.

Nutrition

Fill in your nutrition entries for Day 3.

Sleep

Inspect your bedroom. Is it quiet and restful? If not, change it! You should avoid using your bedroom as a home office where you study, do paperwork or perform other mental chores. Otherwise, as you lie down to sleep, you will be reminded of all the work that remains to be done.

If your bedroom is not in a quiet location, your task for today is to stake out the quietest and most pleasant corner of the room to sleep in. Arrange the position of your bed so that lighting or noise from the street is least disturbing. Substitute low-intensity bedside lamps for any glaring overhead lights.

DAY 4

Affirmation

I will try to exercise today and concentrate on how my body feels while I do it—and on how much better it feels when I am finished.

Keep this statement in mind when you get to the section on exercise, following the section on emotions.

Stress Reduction

Look at the number one "unnecessary stress" in your life. By itself it may not amount to much, but devise a plan to rid yourself of this stress anyway. Perhaps it's something you can delegate—or ignore altogether. (Remember the pie for the office party?) It's worth some thought. The important thing here is to come up with a plan to resolve a specific stress.

Emotions

Remember the wonderful book, speech or movie you reviewed yesterday? Did it inspire you in the same way it did before? If so, why was it so inspirational? How does it relate to your life and your hopes? How can you incorporate what you learned into your everyday life? Take a few minutes to reflect upon this.

Exercise

Today we introduce a new element into the plan: exercise. Many people who suffer from lack of energy find it difficult to even *think* about starting to exercise. But give it a chance; our plan is extremely simple and can be tailored to your individual needs. Working out is especially effective for those whose fatigue is stress induced, for example. So if tension is your problem, you can be more aggressive than the plan suggests. (If you already exercise to some degree, great. Move ahead to match your fitness level.)

On the other hand, people with CFIDS are likely to find that at a certain point, activity will worsen the fatigue, so they must approach exercise cautiously and gently. The plan outlined here is relatively light, but if you notice that your workout makes your fatigue worse or triggers allover muscle aches and flulike symptoms, stay with whatever exercise level you can handle without causing more problems. (See chapter 16 for details.)

For today, think of an exercise that is most appealing and convenient for you, something you visualize yourself doing if you were feeling well and energetic. Review all your options. Are they realistic? You might say you enjoy swimming, but if you don't have ready access to a pool, it's a poor choice.

In this program we're going to use walking as an example because it is always available and cost free. But feel free to substitute your favorite—gardening, tennis, cycling, aerobic dance, whatever. Different personalities are attracted to different activities. I suggest a midmorning workout, if it's practical, but you will be increasing the period to about 45 minutes, so try to allow for that much time at the same time each day. The idea is to emphasize consistency and continuation beyond 30 days; your goal is to establish exercise as a lifelong habit.

Nutrition

Fill in the nutrition entries for Day 4 of your fatigue diary.

Sleep

This might sound silly, but take a good look at your mattress and pillow. Perhaps you've been taking them for granted. Are they really conducive to falling asleep and staying asleep?

The mattress should be firm and large enough so you have room to change positions easily. If your pillow is lumpy (or dusty), throw it out. Today may be an expensive day, but if you need a new mattress and pillow, the purchase is well worth the investment.

DAY 5

Affirmation

Today I will be easy on myself. I will appreciate my many good qualities and not expect more of myself than I am actually capable of doing.

This will help you avoid frustration if you don't see great surges in your energy levels quite yet.

Stress Reduction

How did yesterday go? Did you notice a change in your stress levels? Sometimes the taste of success in removing stress—no matter how small—can be a great motivator in approaching the next part of the task.

Look at the second "unnecessary stress" in your life. Again, formulate a specific plan to deal with it. Explore all your options, and try to think of new ones. As you examine the effects of stress, anticipate the benefits of being relieved of it. As you look at your life from this new perspective, you may want to review your fatigue diary and revise your list of stresses.

Emotions

Today remember a piece of music that had a positive effect on you in the past. Or play a record, tape or CD—preferably something soothing, not exciting, or a number that "sounds" warm and gentle. Listen to the music while you relax or do the stretching exercises described below. Allow the music to lift you and your spirits into a beautiful place.

Exercise

Beginning today and continuing for the next seven days, do some stretching exercises. Start by taking five minutes out of the day, preferably during a low-pressure period that's free of interruptions. (It's a good idea to take the phone off the hook or turn on the answering machine.)

Now sit in your most comfortable chair. First stretch your neck muscles, tilting your head to the left and right, front and back. Lift your arms up over your head, stretching your shoulders and upper back. Raise and lower your arms several times. With your right arm, reach over toward your left elbow to stretch out your chest, shoulder and back muscles a little farther; repeat to the other side. You should feel gentle pressure, but not pain.

Begin moving down your body. Arch your lower back for a slow count of 5, then lean forward slowly, running your hands down your legs. Sit down with your legs out in front of you, then raise one leg and hold it out straight, using your stomach muscles. With your leg still raised, flex your foot, pointing your toes in toward your ankle and stretching the muscles of the calf. Lower and repeat with the left leg.

Next place the ankle of your right leg on your left knee and let your right leg relax. Gently push down on the inside of your right knee, stretching your inner-thigh muscles. Repeat to the other side.

Over the next few days you are going to gradually increase these exercises in number and difficulty so that you will reach all the major muscle groups. But for today and tomorrow, be very gentle. You'll build up slowly to conquer the fatigue.

Try to do your exercises at the same time every day. You are in the process of establishing a routine that you will want to continue after you are feeling better. Exercise should become a lifelong habit to promote, and maintain, vitality and good health.

Nutrition

Continue to fill in the nutrition entries, as described on Day 1.

Sleep

Fine-tune the temperature of your bedroom if it is uncomfortable. Make sure your bedroom isn't too cold and drafty or hot and stuffy. Most people sleep better in a cooler temperature, but be careful to avoid extremes. Experiment with blankets of different weights until you find one that both you and your sleeping partner like.

DAY 6

Affirmation

I will not be stubborn today because I know stubbornness is often a sign of insecurity that can cause me—and others—pain or embarrassment. I have no real reason to feel insecure.

Being flexible and open to ideas helps solutions come more easily.

Stress Reduction

Were yesterday's antistress efforts successful? Did you notice any change at all? If you're not satisfied with your progress, consider these two strategies. You can try again and not move on to the third "unnecessary stress" until the second is resolved. Or, if it turns out that stress number two is simply more intractable than you thought or you're not ready to tackle it, move it farther down on your list and try to work on number three.

Emotions

For the next few days you will attempt to break out of the kinds of ruts that can lead to boredom and apathy. You may not even realize you've gotten into a rut. Today think of a place you always meant to visit but never took the time or energy to do so—a museum, park, aquarium, antique store, hobby shop or friend's house.

Go ahead—do it *today.* Don't let the usual excuses stop you for one more day. If you don't feel well or are very tired, go somewhere quiet where you do not have to walk long distances. And if the place is closed today or your friend isn't home, either make other plans or set a definite time for tomorrow. But get out of the rut of staying at home.

Exercise

Repeat yesterday's gentle stretches for a short time, five minutes or so.

Nutrition

Today review your food diary. How many of your meals, beverages or snacks are heavily sweetened? Is your diet varied, or do you eat pretty much the same thing from day to day? Are you eating any fruit at all? (Fruit is a good source of carbohydrates, potassium and vitamin C, all essential for sufficient energy.) How many times a day do you reach for coffee, tea or cola? (Too much caffeine can rob you of sleep and play havoc with your nerves.)

Another energy-draining pattern to look for is heavy reliance on foods rich in fat: meat, butter, cream, eggs and oil. Remember that cholesterol is found only in animal foods, not in vegetable foods, but fats are found in both groups. A diet that derives a high percentage of calories from fat quickly leads to excess pounds, as we discussed in chapter 14. On a more subjective level, many people report that after cutting down on meat and other animal foods, they feel more energetic. Beginning on Day 8, you will take steps designed to help you cut fat intake without making an abrupt change in your eating habits.

Examine your food diary for any kind of pattern. Most of us are quite repetitive in our eating habits, and our diets probably lean heavily in one direction or another.

At this point, if you don't take vitamin supplements, add a single multiple vitamin to your diet on a daily basis. Choose a good, reputable brand, but not necessarily an expensive one. Ask your pharmacist for advice. The preparation should include essential vitamins along with basic minerals, such as iron, calcium, magnesium and zinc.

Sleep

One of the best ways to cure insomnia is to create a break between the tension of the day and the peacefulness of sleep. So give yourself some time to wind down before climbing into bed, especially if you tend to cram in as much activity as possible before bedtime. Half an hour is ideal. To help yourself relax, read a book or listen to some quiet music. Or tackle some boring correspondence you've been putting off for months. Enjoy a nice warm bath. Measures like these may bring sleep more easily. (If you like to watch television, be sure that your pre-bedtime program won't get your adrenaline going.)

DAY 7

Affirmation

I will do a good deed today. By being nice to someone else, I end up being nice to myself.

See the section on emotions below for the way a good deed can recharge your batteries.

Stress Reduction

Move to the next item on your "unnecessary stress" list, and plan your attack on this one. Is it a deadline? Try to avoid this kind of trap. Think of an approaching deadline and decide if it really counts. If it is neither necessary nor important, don't allow yourself to feel stressed about it. Or change the deadline.

If it *is* important (and deadlines have a tendency to be just that), you may still have some options. Can you get some help to meet it? Can you chuck other obligations to free your time so you can meet this one with less worry and pressure?

One way to deal with a problem that has been causing you stress is to "sleep on it," especially if it's one you feel you must resolve. In other words, you should literally delay your decision until after a good night's sleep; it will reduce your stress. However—and this is very important—don't dwell on the problem while waiting for sleep. Forget it completely. When you wake, you may have a clearer perception of the issues involved. After being cloudy before, the answer or decision may now be obvious.

Emotions

People who are tired all the time get used to staying at home, perpetuating the habit of inactivity. Today, do a good deed. Visit an elderly or disabled friend in a nursing home. Bake a pie for the church social or community fund-raiser. Take some food to a nearby homeless shelter. Sort your clothes and give what you don't wear to the needy. Be sure to write down in your diary how this makes you feel.

Keep in mind, though, that in order for a good deed to have the intended effect, you shouldn't feel pressured into it. And don't feel guilty about the days when you skip helping others.

Exercise

Increase the stretching a little, up to ten minutes, and continue to stretch from a sitting position. Do the same exercises, but put a little more effort into them. If you notice muscle aches, ease up. Then, when the aching has disappeared, advance slowly, at your own pace.

Nutrition

Reread chapter 14, on the link between nutrition and fatigue. Do you have any of the symptoms associated with nutritional deficiency? If you have these in addition to fatigue, examine your nutritional diary to see if you are eating the foods rich in nutrients important to high energy levels.

The best place to start rehabilitating your diet is by cutting down on ice cream, cookies, shakes, soda and any other empty-calorie foods. If you've come to depend on regular sugar "fixes" to get you through the day, try to reduce your intake by at least one-third today, and continue to cut back in this way for the next ten days. You may use a sugar substitute, but it is preferable to reduce the sugar you add to drinks and avoid sugary foods such as sticky buns.

Sleep

If you started out this program by cutting down your dosage of sleep medication, you may now reduce it again by half and maintain this dose for one week. At the same time, continue to wind down for half an hour before bedtime, even if you still do not get to sleep at your "ideal time." The idea is to set a pattern so that when sleep does come at that ideal hour, the pattern will continue long beyond the 30-day period—a godsend for chronic insomniacs.

DAY 8

Affirmation

I do not have to let stress dominate my life. I can choose to react calmly to stressful situations.

In other words, instead of trying to get everything done, focus on remaining calm in the attempt.

Stress Reduction

Move to the fifth "unnecessary stress" on your list. What's your plan? (Review chapter 11 for some useful strategies that work for many people. With trial and error, you begin to learn what works for you and what doesn't.) By now you've probably conquered some minor stress-producing problems and are ready to attack more difficult or important stresses in your life (which presumably follow closely on your list). Perhaps you're involved in a difficult personal relationship or have to deal with an impossible boss or work load, serious financial difficulties or the loss or estrangement of someone close to you.

Today is a good day to evaluate the need for counseling. You have probably observed specific stresses by now, along with your response to them. Take some time to decide if you need professional help. Don't allow shame or guilt to affect your decision. Look at your stresses from a distance to help make up your mind.

If your emotional health is suffering, that's another reason to consider counseling. Are you so depressed that it interferes with your job, your family, your enjoyment of life? As difficult as it may be, try to see yourself objectively, without self-censure. Think of yourself as a friend. What would you tell a friend to do?

Emotions

Do another good deed. Experiment this time—maybe take a risk. When it is done, examine yourself and write about how you feel in your fatigue diary. What does it feel like to help someone? How high was your energy level at the time?

Exercise

Today increase the time you spend stretching to a full ten minutes, stretching from a standing position for half the time. Rotate your trunk from the waist and gently stretch your spine by bending forward. To avoid pressure on the lower back, don't lock your knees or try to touch the floor or your toes. Gently allow gravity to pull your trunk down, but *do not* bounce. If you have CFIDS, be especially careful to avoid straining your back.

Nutrition

Look at the nutrition part of your diary for the first week. How much milk or other diary products do you consume? Milk has been called the perfect food, and it really is—for a growing infant. In my experience, many people with fatigue feel better when they cut down on dairy products. Some researchers claim that it has to do with hidden food allergies, while others cite lactose intolerance. But whatever the cause, try cutting down. Be observant and listen to your body.

If you drink more than one full glass (eight ounces) of milk regularly, try to limit yourself to one glass. You may substitute fruit juices, but if you substitute soda, make it caffeine-free diet soda. At the same time, choose low-fat (1 or 2 percent) milk when you do drink milk. Skim is even better—you get the calcium you need for strong bones, without the fat. An overall reduction of the fat in your diet will improve your energy due to weight reduction, and it will improve the balance of the foods you consume.

Sleep

Continue avoiding caffeine after 5:00 P.M.—no such soft drinks or coffee at supper or afterward. The next step is to drink half as much caffeine-containing beverages during the day. Either make fewer trips to the coffee machine or dilute each cupful with decaffeinated. Continue this for the next week.

If you take nap breaks instead of coffee breaks, heed this: Some people need to nap more, some less. Much depends on how long you nap.

If you take long naps during the day, try to cut down. Daytime naps are among the most important contributors to insomnia. Refer back to your fatigue journal and look at the pattern of daytime naps. For the next week, eliminate half of the daytime sleeping. That is, if you take two hour-long naps during the day, take only one for the next week. If you take only one hour-long nap, make it 30 minutes.

In contrast, you may take "power naps"; that is, naps while sitting that last no more than five to ten minutes. These very short entrances into sleep can be amazingly refreshing and usually do not contribute to insomnia. In fact, if you suffer from insomnia and do not nap during the day, no matter how tired you feel, an occasional short nap may be just what you need.

Note: If you frequently nod off unintentionally at inappropriate times (at an important meeting, while driving the car or in the middle of a conversation), ask your doctor to check you for narcolepsy.

DAY 9

Affirmation

Tonight I will give myself enough time to unwind from the day's stresses and activities to make sure that when I go to bed I will be ready to go to sleep.

Stress Reduction

Take a couple of days to evaluate how successfully you jettisoned the first five mini-stresses. Over the next day or two, finish off any of these five that are not resolved. If you were successful, do you notice a difference now? If you weren't successful, try to understand why not.

Emotions

Today's emotional exercise is the exact opposite of the ones for the past two days: Take 15 minutes (but no more) and feel sorry for yourself. Don't go out, don't do anything; just think about the unfairness of life and the misery of your situation, your bad luck. Pay attention to what it does to your mood and your energy levels. It's like pulling the plug, right? Take out your diary and jot down a few lines about how you feel.

The point of this exercise is to compare how you felt after the good deed yesterday and how you felt after wallowing in self-pity today. What does the self-pity do? What did it get you? Experience this and learn from it.

Exercise

Continue to stretch for ten minutes every day. At this point you may want to choose a sunny, well-lit room along with some soothing music for your routine. Relax, and don't worry about how you're doing. Exercise can help in reducing stress, but not if it's stressful in itself.

Nutrition

If you eat eggs, cut down. Eggs are not only very high in cholesterol, their ratio of protein to fat is not as healthy as in other foods. (A certain amount of protein is essential to adequate energy levels.) Thanks to the availability of cholesterol-free substitutes, most people can still enjoy "eggs." Attempt to reduce your overall egg consumption by at least half.

Sleep

Today's goal is to continue reducing nighttime stimuli. Beginning today, increase the time you spend winding down before bedtime from half an hour to an hour.

DAY 10

Affirmation

Today I will reduce any stress that comes my way by facing troublesome situations with strength, courage and determination.

Stress Reduction

Think of a stress that you will face today, one that you cannot escape. Think of it as a task that must be accomplished or an intriguing jigsaw puzzle you've found in the attic. Resolve to face it bravely and with strength. That will reduce any stress associated with it.

Emotions

Make a "gratitude list" in your diary today. List everything you are grateful for: the fact that you are alive, you have a roof over your head, you have food, you have friends who like to go out to lunch with you or get together and play cards, you have healthy children and so forth.

Take 15 minutes and list everything you can think of. As you regain energy and feel better about yourself, the gratitude list begins to grow because your ability to feel gratitude grows.

Exercise

At midmorning do your usual ten minutes of stretching.

Nutrition

Fats are "heavy foods." Remember how you felt after the last heavy meal you ate? Many people describe a feeling of exhaustion or being drained after a fatty meal, as the body tried to digest its burden. Conversely, countless people report that they feel considerably more energetic after adopting a low-fat diet. So today, and for the rest of the days in this program, trim all fat off meats. Substitute steamed or broiled fish, skinless chicken or turkey for beef and pork—or buy the leaner loin-end cuts. Chances are you won't enjoy your meals any less, but the amount of fat you consume is certain to drop. Simply reducing fats may also help you trim off pounds—which means less excess weight to carry around like a ball and chain every day.

Sleep

Think of a hobby that you have always wanted to take up but just never took the time for—maybe piano playing or wood carving. Consider incorporating it into your wind-down period. It should be an activity that does not overstimulate you but takes your mind off the day's routines.

Don't be too ambitious—otherwise your hobby could become yet another form of pressure. In fact, if it serves its purpose, you won't accomplish much because as you begin work on it, you should get sleepy. So much for becoming a concert pianist.

DAY 11

Affirmation

I will spend time today exercising my skills for communicating by sharing my feelings with another person.

Stress Reduction

Take a deep breath: Today you will focus on a major stress in your life—perhaps not the most important one on the list, but one that really counts. Write it down in your diary, and list the reasons why it is stressful—it makes you angry, hurt or resentful, it wastes time, it makes you tired and so on. Then write down every option you can think of for dealing with this stress.

Emotions

For the next few days you will work to improve your mood by improving communication. Most people have trouble with interpersonal communication, but for some it is a major contributor to depression. Many people who suffer from fatigue tend to become isolated, further hampering communication.

Today think about how you communicate with others. Are you a "yeller"? A "sulker"? Are you expressive of your emotions, or do you hide them? Do you show anger? Are you afraid of anger? How do you show it? Are you the silent type who feels insulted when people do not understand your intentions? Note your style in your diary. And don't forget to describe the kinds of conversations you have with friends, family and co-workers. Are they calm, rational discussions? Monosyllabic exchanges? Long, analytical consultations? Be specific.

Exercise

Today be a little more vigorous; do all the stretches while standing. Also, don't time yourself. Decide when to stop based upon how you feel. You may find that you can comfortably work out for 15 or 20 minutes without realizing it. (Remember, we're working up to 45 minutes.)

Nutrition

Check on the cheeses in your diet. Although these dairy products have some excellent nutritional assets—namely, protein and calcium—they also tend to be high in fat. Where possible, use nonfat cottage cheese, mozzarella or other fat-free cheese products instead of full-fat cheeses, including cream cheese and Brie.

Unless your doctor advises otherwise, you may want to consider adding a single vitamin C supplement to your daily diet. Many Americans are low in vitamin C, and several studies indicate that this nutrient may improve overall health and reduce the risk of cancer. Some researchers advocate its use in CFIDS as a specific treatment because of its antioxidant properties—that is, it scavenges waste products of oxygen metabolism known as free radicals, which are associated with premature cell damage and heart disease. A daily supplement of 500 milligrams of vitamin C is considered modest and safe.

Sleep

Look over your fatigue diary and examine the pattern of your sleep difficulties. If you're still lying awake too long after you go to bed, decide what time you would like to fall asleep and note it in your fatigue diary. Maybe you'd like to get to sleep at 11:00 every night, but you rarely go to bed before midnight and it takes you until at least 1:00 A.M. to fall asleep.

To reset your "sleep clock," move your bedtime a half hour closer to your "ideal sleep time" and continue this for the next few days.

DAY 12

Affirmation

Today I will give someone a big hug and enjoy being physically close to someone I care about.

Stress Reduction

Take some concrete steps toward resolving the major stress you decided yesterday to tackle. If, like most stresses, it's not taken care of quickly and easily, take several days to test different options.

Meanwhile, plan now to take a day off in the next week or so. Decide what is a good day and make it a holiday. There must be a time when you can arrange for someone to watch the children or when you are not needed at work. Feel free to loaf and pamper yourself. Your stress level will plummet, and when you return to active duty, you'll feel amazingly refreshed.

Emotions

Let someone you love know how you feel. Give that person a big hug today—out of the blue. Enjoy it; don't be afraid and don't be embarrassed. If the person asks why the hug, say you just wanted to do it. Allow yourself to feel the warmth of the embrace, and let it lift your mood. If it is not returned, don't be upset. Try it again tomorrow. Pretty soon you'll get a hug, too.

If you don't feel comfortable with this kind of spontaneous expression of feeling, don't worry about it. Not everyone feels natural giving or receiving a hug. Some people simply aren't raised in demonstrative families. If you are not expressive in this way, look for some other suitable way to express your affection—a friendly note of appreciation to someone you work with, perhaps. For similar reasons, choose your subject carefully. But remember, it needs to be clear and open communication.

Exercise

Repeat yesterday's activity.

Nutrition

Iron is essential to prevent iron-deficiency anemia, a commonly diagnosed cause of fatigue. So add a little natural iron to your diet. For a snack, try a portion of raisins, perhaps one of those small snack boxes. Since iron isn't always absorbed efficiently, you want to be sure to eat fruit (like citrus fruit or cantaloupe) on a daily basis—it provides vitamin C, which aids iron absorption.

Keep an eye on your iron intake. With daily vitamin supplementation and a balanced diet, you should be getting plenty of iron, but it's good to make sure. While much of your iron is recycled internally, you normally excrete at least 3 milligrams, sometimes more, daily. Cellular immune responses are decreased when iron is low, and this should be a concern for those with CFIDS. Of course, excessive iron intake can cause problems, too, so don't overdo it. Iron in meats is better absorbed than that in vegetables. Your hemoglobin level should be at least 12 grams.

DAY 13

Affirmation

I will take a walk today and enjoy feeling physically tired and mentally revitalized when I am through.

Stress Reduction

This is the second day of attacking the major stress you chose.

Emotions

Communicate with those you love. Think of something you really like about someone you care for and find the opportunity to share your feelings. Perhaps you can compliment someone at work on a job well done. Maybe your mate remembered to take care of an errand or chore around the house, and you want to express your thanks. If your husband or wife lost a few pounds or bought a new outfit, be sure to express your admiration.

Focus on a special trait in a loved one and show that person how much you admire this quality.

Exercise

Today you move on from the stretching exercises and begin walking. It's an ideal exercise that incorporates every muscle group. It will tone the muscles, aid digestion, burn calories and reduce stress. It's perfect for stress reduction because it is difficult to concentrate on life's worries while walking.

Plan your route, starting with one that will take about ten minutes. Think about going through your neighborhood, a nearby park or some attractive place that you pass as you drive to work. Wear comfortable, loose clothing and well-broken-in sneakers (a new pair may cause blisters). Better yet, wear running or walking shoes—footwear specifically designed for athletic activity; they give more support than canvas sneakers. Acrylic socks (not cotton) also help prevent friction.

Make your first walk slow and easy.

Nutrition

Now that you've cut energy-sapping fat from your diet, it's time to check for any food sensitivities you might have. It takes some experimentation to see how your body reacts to certain foods. For today, try eating a larger amount of dairy products than usual (particularly since you cut the amount in the past ten days). If you are sensitive to these foods, you might notice fatigue, bloating and abdominal gas. Such a response tells you to cut way back on dairy products in the future. You may want to add Lactaid (an enzyme product that helps in digesting milk solids) to see if it eases your reaction to dairy products, particularly abdominal bloating or gas.

DAY 14

Affirmation

Today I will spend some time nourishing my personal growth by opening myself up in a long letter to someone I care about but haven't seen or heard from in a long time.

Stress Reduction

Were you successful in disposing of the major stress you chose? If so, you should be aware of a pronounced difference in your life. Stresses are not hopeless pits of quicksand that lie in front of you. They are problems that can be approached by rational planning. They can be resolved (albeit some more easily than others).

Emotions

Communicate with old friends, perhaps people you have not seen in years. Call them up or write a letter. Tell them that you miss them; expose your feelings, even take a few risks. Make sure they know how you feel.

Exercise

Take another ten-minute walk. While you may have heard that a brisk, fast walk is better exercise than a relaxed, gentle one, stay with your slower pace for now. The purpose of the walk is to break the cycle of anxiety as well as tone the muscles. You want to associate exercise with relaxation and enjoyment, not exhaustion and stress.

Nutrition

Look over your diet record and count how many servings of vegetables you ate. (Potato chips and onion rings don't count.) The diet eaten by many Americans (at least until lately) has been too rich in fats and too short on vegetables. Try to build up the vegetable side of your daily menu.

Leafy vegetables are wonderful sources of nutrients like iron, folate and magnesium, essential to keeping energy levels from flagging. They also contribute some calcium and vitamins E and K. Magnesium is particularly important for people plagued with fatigue, so be sure your diet contains those greens, plus other sources such as broccoli and beans. They're also low in fat and calories and high in fiber.

Have at least one good-sized helping of vegetables at your main meal every day. And don't stick to the same few choices. Eat a different one every day. To avoiding depleting nutrients, never overcook the vegetables. (Another reason a microwave can be a boon to weary cooks: It saves time *and* keeps the green beans from fading to khaki.)

Sleep

If you're still taking a measurable dose of a sedative tablet, cut the dose in half again and maintain this for a week. At the same time, halve the amount of caffeine that you've been drinking daily over the past week. Or switch to decaf entirely. Either way, continue this for another week.

DAY 15

Affirmation

Today I will take a mental, physical and spiritual inventory. I will review my daily journal and be happy with what I have accomplished and what I have learned in the past two weeks. I will also resolve to do even more by making full use of my talents.

Stress Reduction

Today's task is to set some kind of goal for yourself. Think about something definite you would like to accomplish this week, this month or this year, and make it your specific aim. Be sure it's practical and can be reasonably achieved—not too difficult a task, nor one that will add to your stress. In fact, the goal should help reduce your stress and allow you to feel good about your accomplishment.

Think in terms of starting a small garden, meeting a new neighbor or lunching with an old friend.

Emotions

Reach out to a friend by sending a gift or flowers. You don't need a specific reason; you're just saying that you care. There are many ways besides words to communicate. The most meaningful messages come by way of the actions of love. You might want to buy a stack of pretty postcards and prestamp them, so you can jot down a few words to old friends throughout the year. (This serves two purposes: It helps prevent isolation, and it helps cut down on the dread of having to write long, personal greetings on each and every Christmas card you send out, reducing holiday stress and burnout.)

Exercise

By now you have decided on the best time of day to exercise—first thing in the morning, after breakfast, midmorning, during your lunch break or after work. Don't schedule exercise near bedtime because it may stimulate your adrenaline and make getting to sleep more difficult. You will be adding some pre-bedtime stretching after the walks become more vigorous.

Nutrition

To continue to investigate possible food sensitivities, try eating an abundance of fruit today. Have a big salad consisting of several varieties of fresh fruit. It's rare, but some people can't tolerate fructose, the principal sugar in fruits. For them nausea, gas and sometimes vomiting will follow a fructose overload. In others the blood sugar level drops after a fructose-rich meal.

If you don't feel well after a eating a large portion of fruit, it's possible that you are sensitive to fructose and should limit the amount of fruit you eat at any one time.

Add a small portion (perhaps ½ cup) of unsalted nuts to your diet. You might have them as a snack, one that you can carry with you on your walk. Nuts are rich in protein and minerals. But don't go overboard—nuts are high in fat and calories. (And of course, don't try this if you have a known allergy to nuts.)

Otherwise continue to strive for a diet rich in starchy foods like potatoes, rice and pasta, plenty of vegetables and a moderate amount of low-fat protein—all conducive to good energy reserves.

Sleep

Continue to keep track of how much sleep you get at night and any naps you take during the day.

Also, if you aren't getting to bed on time, make an extra effort to move toward your ideal sleep time. Now you also begin to shift your wake-up time. Many individuals who have insomnia fall asleep late and compensate by sleeping longer in the morning. To be successful in adjusting the sleep clock, you need to move the wake-up time as well. If you move your bedtime a half hour earlier, be sure also to get up a half hour earlier in the morning. Maintain this bedtime for five days.

DAY 16

Affirmation

Tonight when I go to bed, I will be eager to fall asleep. I will enjoy a good night's rest and wake up refreshed in the morning.

Stress Reduction

Begin working toward the goal you set. Be gentle and kind to yourself, but approach the goal with firmness and assurance.

Emotions

Contact a friend or loved one you admire, perhaps someone you have not seen in a while. Communication tends to be a little harder with family than with friends, so if you decide to get in touch with a long-lost relative, congratulate yourself on establishing a new tie.

Exercise

Remember to take your walk today, again for about ten minutes. You may want to take a different route or walk in a new location, preferably with sunshine and greenery, to expand your horizons. My favorite routes are paths through woods because I love to listen to songbirds. As it so happens, my coauthor enjoys walking, too!

Nutrition

Review your everyday diet, catalogued in the first five days of the program. Did you eat any fish or seafood? It would be an excellent substitute for some of the meat in your menu—at least once a week.

Certain types of fish, such as cod, haddock and flounder, are excellent sources of protein with relatively little fat. But even oilier species such as tuna, mackerel and salmon have potential benefits. One medical study of people with CFIDS found that fish-oil supplements improved energy levels and reduced the degree of fatigue. While there are many possible explanations, the improvement could have been due to the overall balance of the fatty acids eaten or to replenishing the body's stores of certain essential fatty acids deficient in the diet.

Sleep

Now it's off to sleep with a technique called sleep visualization. Its purpose is to simultaneously relax the body and turn off the mind. As you practice this over the next two weeks, you'll become more proficient, and it should take less time for you to fall asleep. Your ultimate goal is to fall asleep within 30 seconds of beginning the technique, but don't pressure yourself or it might not work at all.

Start by getting comfortable in bed. Beginning with your scalp muscles and moving down your body, you'll learn, muscle group by muscle group, to visualize how the muscles feel when completely relaxed. Move from your head to your face and neck, then your arms, legs and so forth—sort of like layers of limp lasagna. You will notice that when you visualize each muscle relaxed, it will actually relax, almost magically.

For tonight spend three or four minutes practicing this technique on your face muscles only.

DAY 17

Affirmation

Today I will make peace with someone I have problems with. Whether they are willing to make peace with me has nothing to do with my decision to try to resolve our difficulties. I am responsible for my feelings toward them, not their feelings toward me.

Stress Reduction

Once again, pay close attention to any signs of stress you may be experiencing, like sweaty palms or rapid heartbeat. If you detect these symptoms during the day, rather than allow the stress to continue, take a time-out and talk with someone, listen to music or take a bath. Don't allow the stress to consume you.

Emotions

Today's "emotional calisthenic" is a little tougher. Contact a relative with whom you have had some difficulty. (If you've had no such difficulty, congratulations on your good fortune.) If you've had an argument, apologize and ask that whatever angry words you might have said be forgiven. Express yourself honestly, but do try to mend the broken fence. Today's is a difficult task, one that most of us are afraid to undertake. But unresolved conflicts can drag you down, weighing heavily on your spiritual energy. So what can you lose? If your relative does not forgive you, at least you tried. Feel good about your attempt and your growing powers of communication!

Exercise

Today walk a little longer—15 or 20 minutes, but keep the pace easy.

Nutrition

Ten days ago you reduced your sugar intake by about a third. Reduce it again by another third or even half. This should cut your consumption of candy or other sweets (including soda, and sugar added to tea or coffee) considerably. There's no need to avoid all desserts. It's not your aim to eliminate every bit of sugar, just to reduce the amount you use, in case excessive sugar contributes to your fatigue.

Sleep

Today's sleep tip is related to diet. Try a few natural foods that may help to soothe you as an overture to sleep. At your evening meal, include foods that are relatively high in the amino acid tryptophan, such as low-fat milk, cheese, chicken and turkey. Some evidence suggests that tryptophan is a natural sleep inducer, and an evening meal or snack high in this amino acid serves as an overture to sleep. One caution, however: Don't rely on commercial preparations of tryptophan, which were taken off the market a few years ago because of hazards of contamination. Natural food sources are safer.

DAY 18

Affirmation

I am powerless over much of what happens to me, but I can control how I react to it. Today I will face life armed with a sense of humor—one of life's most valuable coping tools.

Stress Reduction

Theologians and medical researchers alike find that religious beliefs give people a blueprint for life that helps them better cope with daily stresses and improve their overall outlook. So today take a step toward some kind of spiritual growth and exploration. Start by defining your own spiritual views. Do you believe in God? Do you believe that there are forces outside of yourself that are important, even though they may not be easily recognized? Do you believe that these forces have spiritual value? Would you like to explore the spiritual nature of existence?

During tough times, many people return to the spiritual belief system (i.e., religion) of their childhood for guidance. Or perhaps you've been meaning to explore a new denomination or belief system. Now is a good time to do so.

Take a few minutes in a quiet place to think about these matters.

Emotions

Communicate some of your deep feelings to a friend. Perhaps share an inner secret, worry or fear. Take a risk by expressing yourself to someone you trust. If that's not convenient, open up to your diary and try to put your concerns on paper. Studies by James W. Pennebaker, Ph.D., at Southern Methodist University in Dallas, indicate that people who find a way to divulge their innermost thoughts and feelings find it easier to resolve those feelings. The effect is therapeutic.

Exercise

Once again, take a 15- or 20-minute walk. And again, try a new place. (If it's raining or cold, go to a nearby mall.)

Nutrition

Researchers have noted that people with headaches (especially migraine-type headaches) tend to suffer fatigue. Many migraine sufferers are also sensitive to certain foods, like aged cheese, chocolate, cured meats and monosodium glutamate. Other researchers report that many people with CFIDS experience headaches after eating certain foods. Either way, identifying and avoiding trigger foods may help restore energy levels.

If you suffer any kind of headache, try to trace the pain to what you eat for the next ten days, using your fatigue diary.

You may also want to avoid all wheat in your diet today. That means no breads, cookies or pasta. Some people are sensitive to wheat and will have abdominal distress and excessive fatigue after eating it. If you are not sure of your response to any of these food-sensitivity tests, experiment further. Observe the responses that certain foods evoke in you, and adjust your diet accordingly.

Sleep

Tonight concentrate again on relaxing your body and turning off your mind. Begin by visualizing the relaxation of your scalp muscles and feeling them go limp, even the tiny ones under your hair. Move to the jaw muscles and the muscles around your ears. Feel them fall into place. Relax your tongue. When you do, you'll experience the odd sensation of having to figure out where to rest your tongue. Suddenly, wherever you put it seems awkward. Rest it somewhere behind your teeth, where it should be comfortable, and move on to the muscles of your face and neck. (This interesting phenomenon makes you realize how much energy you spend on little things that you never think about.) You will soon fall asleep.

DAY 19

Affirmation

Today I will spend some time by myself meditating. I will explore my personal spiritual development and concentrate on the role a higher power can play in enhancing my life.

Stress Reduction

Today's tension reliever is rooted in spiritual practices of various religions. Take a few minutes to meditate.

Find a quiet place and take time to become relaxed and comfortable. Focus your thoughts on spiritual matters you considered yesterday. Concentrate on what direction in spiritual learning you would like to go.

Perhaps you've had a bad experience involving spiritual matters—a disillusioning incident, a falling out with a member of your church or synagogue or a rigid, disciplined religious upbringing that took the joy out of your spiritual life. Whatever may have happened, try to start again. Think about meditation as a way to calm yourself and quiet your soul.

Emotions

If someone has been offensive to you, communicate your displeasure to them. Express it clearly but not harshly. Perhaps you might say something such as "I understand why you . . . , but I feel . . . " or "I feel angry about. . . " The point is to make your communication clear, so that the other person understands. If you are angry, it's okay to say so. The trick is to say it calmly. Most of us are afraid to express our anger, yet when we do, it clears the air like a thunderstorm on a hot and humid day. Otherwise our anger smolders and feeds on our energy reserves, robbing us not only of energy but of the joy in life.

Exercise

Before you take your walk today, warm up for five minutes by jogging in place. Then stretch your leg and shoulder muscles—do a few ankle rotations or windmills with your arms. By gearing up your muscles and revving up your blood circulation, you'll notice that you walk a little faster, and the chance of muscle strain is reduced. Plus, you'll be more relaxed from the start.

From today on your walk will become more vigorous, so get into the habit of warming up.

Nutrition

Now is a good time to reassess your daily intake of fruit. If you don't seem to have any sensitivity to fruit, apricots, peaches, berries, melons, bananas and so forth are excellent sources of vitamins, minerals and complex carbohydrates as well as dietary fiber. Try to add at least one fruit to your customary diet. But don't eat the same one or two every day. A variety helps to ensure that you will avail yourself of all the nutrients various fruits have to offer. Fresh fruit is preferable to that canned in syrup. Dried fruit is convenient to keep on hand, especially if you don't have the energy to make your weekly excursion to the store.

At this point it's also a good idea to increase your dietary fiber by substituting whole-grain breads and bran cereals for white bread and rice or refined cereals. Many Americans are deficient in thiamine, a B vitamin present in the part of wheat that's usually discarded in processing white flour. Plus, getting a daily quota of 20 to 30 grams of fiber can help prevent constipation, often associated with feelings of overall sluggishness. But you'll want to increase your fiber intake gradually to avoid intestinal distress.

Sleep

Scientific studies show that excessive alcohol consumption causes reduced magnesium levels, and adequate magnesium is essential for energy. Even a few casual beers after work or a glass or two of wine with dinner can sap daytime energy levels without your realizing it. And as noted in chapter 17, steady consumption of beer, wine or liquor on a regular basis interferes with the quality of your sleep. So if you drink, cut your alcohol intake by half. If you drink alcohol *and* use sleep medications, this reduction is a very important step toward improving your sleep. Better yet, try to do without your customary alcohol intake.

If you're exceptionally sensitive to alcohol, this is strongly suggestive of CFIDS; very few persons with CFIDS drink at all because of how it affects them.

In addition, move further with your visualization. You will notice that it becomes easier to relax certain muscles the second or third time around. As you gain proficiency at this and other relaxation techniques, you should be able to rely less and less on alcohol or sleep aids to help you unwind and fall asleep.

DAY 20

Affirmation

I will appreciate a friend today and be thankful for the many joys that friendship brings to my life. I will also tell that friend just how much he or she means to me.

Stress Reduction

Begin a more formalized technique for meditation.

Option 1: You might read a few lines from an inspirational book and allow your thoughts to focus upon that as you meditate. Take a thought and allow it to drift through your consciousness. Don't try to solve anything. Relax.

Option 2: If prefer to pursue a more directed approach with specific religious instructions, substitute them here. Prayer can be tremendously healing for both the soul and the body. But don't pretend you feel something that's not there. It is of no value and may eat away at any gains you've made.

Whichever option you choose, find a quiet but comfortable area in your home and choose a time that is pressure free. Sit in a comfortable position, but with your back straight. You do not want to be so comfortable that you fall asleep; that exercise is for later in the evening.

Allow your mind to roam without structure. Relax your muscles and give yourself ten minutes for healing and renewal.

Emotions

Today try to improve some aspect of interpersonal communication.

Option 1: If you feel up to it, think of a relationship that's causing some sort of distress—perhaps a situation that is marred by hopeless communication with someone you just cannot get across to. Talk with that person and attempt to straighten it out. Give it a try; take a risk. If it works out, good. If it remains hopeless, compliment yourself on the attempt. Remember that communication is a two-way street, and you are responsible only for your way.

Option 2: If you can't handle a confrontation right now, call a friend and go for a walk. (Combine two steps into one!)

Exercise

Repeat yesterday's workout.

Nutrition

Again, increase dietary fiber by being sure your diet contains such foods as beans, broccoli, cauliflower and Swiss chard. Leafy green vegetables are smart choices, too—they add beta-carotene and fiber.

Sleep

If you're still using some form of sleep aid, take your present dose every other night (rather than nightly) for the rest of the week. Meanwhile, if you're still not falling asleep as expected, try once again to reset your sleep clock. Move your bedtime another half hour toward your ideal sleep time. Remember to move your wake-up time by the same amount. If you are now retiring at the ideal time, stay here until the close of the 30 days. If you are still off, maintain this bedtime for 5 days.

DAY 21

Affirmation

Today I will walk a little farther than on Day 13. Instead of thinking about all the problems or challenges I face, I will use the time to be thankful for all the blessings in my life and the power within me to handle whatever comes my way.

Stress Reduction

Practice your chosen form of meditation again today.

Emotions

Take a few moments to reflect on your experiments in communication over the past ten days. Think of what you tried and what happened as a result. Remember how you felt when you attempted new forms of communication. How did this communication affect your attitudes? Make some notes in your diary because you may want to remind yourself in the future of what was probably the energizing effect of clear, warm and direct communication.

Exercise

Today walk for a full 25 minutes. Choose another area, since you will cover a little more territory. Just be sure the place is safe. It will not ease your anxiety if you walk where you're in danger of being mugged!

Nutrition

Today's the big day: It's now time to eliminate caffeine altogether. If you enjoy the taste of coffee, substitute decaffeinated coffee, but consume only a small amount. Even without the caffeine, the association of coffee with the jitters can bring back anxiety and sleeplessness. Maintain a caffeine-free diet for the remainder of the 30-day program—perhaps for the rest of your life, if it seems to help.

Sleep

As you begin your visualization tonight, concentrate deeply, but not so hard that you get anxious. Relax the muscles of your chest, and picture your heart muscles themselves relaxing down to the individual fibers. With practice, you may notice your heart rate dropping when you do this.

DAY 22

Affirmation

I will examine my mood today—good or bad. I will try to understand why I feel the way I do and what could have triggered it. Then I will decide if I want to continue to feel this way and what to do if I choose to change.

Stress Reduction

Talk with a friend who has spiritual views you never really discussed in full. Try to hear what he or she is saying. Don't react defensively if the views are different from your own. Listen openly. You do not have to agree. If there is even one sentence your friend says that is true or interesting, store it in your memory for further reflection. Don't be afraid if you hear something of Truth; it often comes in unexpected packages.

Observe how you feel after the discussion. Are you angry? Uplifted? How is your energy level? Try to understand your feelings as a result of the discussion.

Emotions

Examine your mood today. Are you depressed? If so, what set it off? Try to pinpoint associations between your moods and specific events. Is your mood related to communication with specific people? To menses? To the anniversary of a loved one's death?

Most of us don't realize that our moods are linked to specific events that might trigger depression. Just seeing that the associations exist allows us to cope better and may even eliminate depression.

Exercise

Think about your favorite walking location, and use a map to find other places you might enjoy as well. Don't ignore the beautiful areas within a short drive of your home.

Nutrition

Cut down on your salt intake by adding less and reducing your consumption of salty foods such as pretzels, corn chips and potato chips by at least half. If you miss these snack foods, try substituting unsalted popcorn. A large amount of salt requires large volumes of fluids to help pass it through the kidneys. Sometimes people eat such high amounts of salted foods that they drink excessive amounts of fluid, and that can disturb the concentration of nutrients in the bloodstream, causing or adding to fatigue.

Sleep

To help you unwind before bedtime, make yourself a cup of hot herbal tea, a kind without caffeine or stimulants. My particular favorite is chamomile. Not only is the tea itself soothing, the act of preparing it is soothing and relaxing as well.

As you perform your sleep visualization tonight, concentrate on your legs. Restless legs syndrome is a very unpleasant cause of insomnia. Try to relax those muscles thoroughly. You may notice that relaxing them feels strange until you get used to it. But relaxed muscles conserve energy, so you'll fall asleep more quickly. (Your bed partner will get more rest, too, if you're less prone to twitching and jerking in your sleep.) You can even visualize a switch intended to keep the muscles relaxed for a prolonged period.

DAY 23

Affirmation

Today I will set aside some time for laughter. Maybe I'll rent a comedy and watch it on my VCR, read a funny book or remember and relive the last time I had a really good, long laugh.

Stress Reduction

Meditate again today, and let yourself drift into a deeper state of relaxation than yesterday. (But try not to fall asleep.) Your mind may stay alert, but it is a gentle, relaxed alertness.

Emotions

You've heard that laughter is good medicine. Make sure you get your share. Think of a movie that was hilariously funny to you. Rent it and watch it early this evening. Allow yourself to laugh and laugh and laugh.

Exercise

Today walk slowly and enjoy the scenery: Savor the taste of fresh air, the sounds of nature, the smell of flowers. Feel all of you come alive. Forget the pressures that bear down on you. Later you can accomplish everything that needs to get done.

Nutrition

If you don't seem to have any problems with wheat sensitivity, add more cereals. They will increase dietary fiber intake, and they're relatively low in fat. Many persons with fatigue, particularly those with CFIDS, have associated bowel problems. Eating more fiber may be helpful in such a case.

Sleep

By now you should have worked up to a routine where you can use visualization to relax your body, muscle group by muscle group, from head to toe. Once you have relaxed your entire body, you can start again. You will notice that tension built up again in the scalp and jaw muscles after you took your attention off them.

DAY 24

Affirmation

Today I will remind myself that adding fear to pain only makes the pain last longer. Today I will not be afraid.

Stress Reduction

Read a passage or two from an inspirational book of your choice; perhaps the Bible, the Torah or the Koran. Consider spiritual exercises such as yoga. Focus your spiritual energies on something that is consistent with what you truly believe.

Yoga or a similar discipline can be of tremendous value in our lives. Most of us shy away from exploring these disciplines because of unwarranted stereotypes or biases. Consider talking to someone who practices yoga, or go to a class and check it out for yourself. Do not be afraid to experience new things. Many people find that yoga broadens their view of life and benefits their whole body.

If you are reluctant to learn new things about our world, ask yourself why. Perhaps that's a topic for meditation.

Emotions

Today's exercise is for individuals who've struggled with their weight for years and just can't seem to lose those last few pounds. Take 15 minutes and think about it. Don't be critical—you've probably spent years beating yourself up for weight problems. Accept yourself as you are built. Examine your pattern of self-criticism and see how it eats away at your self-esteem and your energy.

Accept an invitation from someone. Go for dinner. Go shopping. Go to the movies. If there are no invitations today, accept the next one you get. Some of us are no longer asked to attend events because the hosts know we always decline. Next time say yes, even if it's for something you're not really keen on. The act of accepting an invitation is a good deed, plus going out breaks you out of your daily routine.

Exercise

Get out and take your 20-minute walk, but walk more vigorously. Swing your arms a little more. Keep your pace steady. (And don't forget your warm-up.)

Nutrition

Now that you've begun an overhaul of your diet, it's time for another five-day record of what you eat. You should be noticing certain differences in your life, not the least of which is an increase in your energy level!

Keeping track of your diet will continue to help you identify links between what you eat and how you feel. But the nutrition portion of your fatigue diary now serves the added purpose of reinforcing the improvements you've made. (You may even begin to call this your *energy* diary.)

Sleep

By now it is likely that your insomnia is much improved and that only a relatively short period of visualization is needed before you drift off.

DAY 25

Affirmation

There are times when I am harder on myself and expect more of myself than anyone else does. If other people treated me the way I sometimes treat myself, I would not tolerate it. Today I will remember to be gentle with myself.

Stress Reduction

Look at the patterns of stress in your life now. Are they different from what they were three weeks ago? Do you recognize the early warning signs of stress? Are you able to manage stress before it begins to build up?

Emotions

Focus on what you have accomplished during the day. Most of us see only our failures and overlook something achieved, something done. Practice looking at the constructive side of your life instead of ignoring it. List your recent accomplishments in your diary.

Exercise

Today increase the length of time you walk, but decrease your speed. No doubt there's been some variation in your exercise period from day to day. It's important for you to be comfortable with that. Take advantage of differences in weather, free time that you might have and how you feel. Experience freedom, but within the constraints of actually doing the exercise. That is, don't feel free to skip your walk.

Nutrition

Continue to keep a record of what you eat and how you feel. Review your day's diet and compare it to the first days of the 30-day program. Is it different? Do you feel good about the changes that you have made?

Sleep

By tonight you should be going to bed at your ideal bedtime and falling asleep soon afterward. If you are still some time away, move to it at this point. Try to maintain your "ideal bedtime." That doesn't mean you have to be inflexible, but the sleep preparations and the associations you are forming will make sleep come more easily, especially if you are consistent. Don't be a slave to habit, but don't become erratic, either. Smoothing the extremes is an effective technique for improving sleep and removing fatigue.

DAY 26

Affirmation

I can feel or imagine the warmth of sunlight and focus on it. In my mind I can see how it fills me with warmth and an inner light. When I meditate, I can sense that inner light spreading to every part of me, and the thought of it gives me peace.

Stress Reduction

Today try to combine your spiritual exercises with your physical exercises. Find a sentence or phrase that holds a spiritual or emotional truth for you. Write it on a piece of paper and take it with you when you walk. Repeat the phrase; memorize it. Allow the phrase to walk with you, and study it. When you finish this exercise, you will have a greater understanding of that truth.

Emotions

Add a little light in the morning to brighten your mood and reestablish the proper daytime alertness and nighttime drowsiness. This advice is based on the observation that light deprivation can alter sleep patterns and induce a type of depression known as seasonal affective disorder.

Try to establish a pattern of exposing yourself to some form of bright daylight in the morning, fading light in the afternoon and relative darkness in the evening.

Option 1: Go outdoors for a few minutes at midmorning. If you chose walking as your exercise, it's best to do it in the morning, not just because of the exercise component, but also because it exposes you to the greatest light intensity.

Option 2: Spend part of the morning in a room in your house with south or southeastern exposure, perhaps a room where you grow houseplants. You may want to spend more time here.

Option 3: Turn on a bright light, especially if it's a gloomy day.

Exercise

Walk for 30 minutes, and remember to warm up first.

Nutrition

Record the third day of your "new" diet in the nutrition section of your fatigue diary. Also, note any changes in your energy level.

Sleep

By now you should no longer need medication to help you fall asleep. The reduction should have been gradual enough so that you barely noticed it when you stopped. The hard part came at the beginning. And from this point on, try to avoid sleep medications, unless your physician directs you to take them.

DAY 27

Affirmation

For today I will recognize the many areas where I have choices in my life. This knowledge will give me freedom, and with my freedom comes joy.

Stress Reduction

Once again, you will be combining the spiritual exercise with the physical. Take the same sentence or phrase that you studied yesterday, but use it to look at things in a new light. As you walk, think about your inspirational phrase as different people or objects catch your eye. In other words, when you see something that gets your attention, look at it "through" the phrase you are repeating. Allow the phrase you are studying to color your understanding of the world around you. You will also notice that your understanding of the meaning or meanings of the phrase will grow. You can't digest it all in one day; there are years of contemplation in it. The only thing required is the drive and motivation to go on thinking about the inspirational idea.

Emotions

Say no to any unnecessary demands made on you. Practice freedom. Allow yourself to decide what you are unwilling to do and to express it clearly. Perhaps it is an extra task at work or a favor someone thinks you owe them. But allow yourself the freedom to say no.

Another way to break out of old, confining habits is to dress differently today. If you always wear serious, businesslike or dark clothes, wear something bright and cheery; if you wear casual, bright clothes, try something conservative. Refuse to be constrained by the habits of the past.

Exercise

Take your daily walk, and don't forget the warm-up.

Nutrition

Record Day 4 of your high-energy diet in your nutrition diary. Is your new eating plan becoming a part of your life?

Sleep

Try the "black hole" visualization. This technique is more advanced and difficult, but it can be very effective and interesting. Doctors, of course, are not immune to insomnia, and when I have trouble falling asleep, I visualize a gently swirling disk, like a thousand stars in a swirling nebula around a black hole in outer space. The center of the disk is the black hole itself, which is sleep and all its mysteries. I visualize the approach to sleep as gently circling and begin farther out if I think that going to sleep will take more than a few seconds. By the time I am close to entering the black hole, I am almost always on the edge of sleep and have occasionally "watched" myself go to sleep. Interesting.

Actually, this technique is similar to other visualizations. It is a process of relaxation and a form of autohypnosis. It breaks the pattern of daytime thoughts that can keep us tossing and turning during the night.

DAY 28

Affirmation

Today I can stretch myself spiritually as well as physically. I can introduce new ideas to my inquiring mind and be open and willing to examine them.

Stress Reduction

Look at some spiritual discipline that you are not familiar with—an eastern belief system like Buddhism, perhaps, or different meditation techniques. Consider it with an open, nonjudgmental mind. Your spiritual values are yours and will not be fundamentally altered by reading something "different." Just by looking into what's unfamiliar, you will learn more about the values that are truly yours.

Emotions

Tell yourself it's okay not to be perfect. Survey the images of perfection you compare yourself to and toss them away. Demand the freedom to be yourself, not some image of perfection that has nothing to do with the reality of who you are. No one is perfect, and none of us will ever be perfect. It's okay to make mistakes, fail or disappoint others from time to time.

Exercise

Choose yet another new area for your walk, perhaps a neighborhood on the other side of town or a trail several miles away. Look on a map for a state park or nature walk, or a museum. This time, don't limit yourself to 30 minutes. In fact, don't time yourself at all; just walk as long as you feel like it. You may notice that you can take a long walk without becoming tired. But do not push it too far over your limits.

Nutrition

Continue to record what you eat. Review your new diet for any obvious imbalance. By now you should be consuming several servings of fruits, vegetables and grains every day, with moderate amounts of dairy products or meat and a minimal reliance on fats and sweets.

Sleep

If the sleep techniques described here work for you, continue to make them a part of your nightly routine. But if you still have difficulty getting to sleep and staying asleep, maybe you should be evaluated in a sleep laboratory. You can ask your own physician for a referral, or call the main desk of any large referral hospital for information. If you have not responded despite diligent attempts, a sleep specialist may offer specific therapy for your particular condition.

Even if you need medical advice for a sleep problem, the exercises in this program will put you a step ahead. The sleep specialist might prescribe some of these same suggestions.

DAY 29

Affirmation

Friendship is a precious gift that is freely given to such fortunates as me. It has no price. It is beyond value. Today I will focus some energy on being a friend to one who is in special need of my friendship.

Stress Reduction

Meditate again today, and think about your long-term spiritual goals. Focus on what you would like to learn, what you would like to try. Is existence merely physical? Is there such a thing as the Spirit, a higher power of some kind? Formulate a plan for approaching these questions in a relaxed manner over the next few months. Set a goal for yourself, one that is achievable.

Emotions

Think of a good deed that is above and beyond the call of duty, perhaps a more difficult task; maybe something that requires sacrifice on your part. A good deed that no one you know would do. Give it a try. Expend whatever energy you have today doing something that will help someone else. Act in such a way that no one knows you were the one who did it. You are not trying to earn a compliment. See how it feels.

Exercise

Take your walk again today, anywhere you please. But ask a friend to go with you. Modify your walk to your friend's pace, but don't go beyond what you can comfortably do. Enjoy the companionship. (If none of your friends are available today, offer to walk their dog.)

Nutrition

Take a look at the pattern of your daily diet now, compared with when you began the program. Is your diet more balanced? Has the amount of sugar and fat you consume decreased? Has alcohol intake been drastically reduced or eliminated? Have you noticed food sensitivities? Are the types of protein you eat now (lean meat, more poultry and fish) as satisfying as what you ate before (fatty beef and pork)? Do you eat enough leafy vegetables, complex carbohydrates and fruit for the magnesium, vitamin C and other nutrients necessary for energy?

Your new diet should be healthier without causing suffering or anguish. Make notes in your diary to summarize the changes you made. In the future, if you notice the fatigue returning, refer to this diary for reminders of those revisons and how they affected your energy level.

DAY 30

Affirmation

Today I will celebrate my increased energy and be grateful for the magnificent changes the last 30 days have made in my life. I will also carry on with my physical, emotional and spiritual programs so I can continue to have even more energy and enjoy the inner power I feel in using it.

Take stock of the various areas of your life you've been working on over the past month—stress reduction, emotional harmony, physical stamina, better nutrition and sounder sleep.

Perhaps a repeat visit to your doctor is in order to repeat your tests for cholesterol and triglyceride levels. (They should be lower.) Your blood pressure should be improved, too. Ask your doctor for his or her impression of how you look. Better or the same? Is there a change in your weight? In your attitude? Do you communicate better? Do you feel less stressed?

Now for the critical question: Do you feel better? Do you have more energy? Grade your overall energy level from 0 (none) to 10 (full of vitality), using the same measures as you did on Day 1 of the program. Is it improved?

Most people need time to incorporate changes in their lifestyle. Don't be discouraged if you did not accomplish all you intended to. You may have made some changes, and you are now healthier because of it. Maybe you can do more in the next 30 days.

You certainly know more now about how your body responds than you did before beginning the program. Use what you have learned to set your goals for the coming weeks and months. Make notes to yourself.

Your first 30 days are up, but your lifelong program is just beginning. Good luck!

Index